EVIDENCE-BASED MEDICINE

How to practice and teach it

FOURTH EDITION

Sharon E. Straus

Professor, Department of Medicine, University of Toronto, St Michael's Hospital, Toronto, Ontario, Canada

Paul Glasziou

Director, Centre for Evidence-Based Practice, University of Oxford, Oxford, UK

W. Scott Richardson

Professor of Medicine, and Campus Associate Dean for Curriculum, MCG/UGA Medical Partnership Campus, Athens, Georgia, USA

R. Brian Haynes

Professor of Clinical Epidemiology and Medicine, McMaster University, Hamilton, Ontario, Canada

CHURCHILL LIVINGSTONE

ELSEVIER

Edinburgh London New York Oxford Philadelphia St Louis Sydney Toronto 2011

CHURCHILL
LIVINGSTONE
ELSEVIER

First edition 1997, Second edition 2000, Third edition 2005, Fourth edition 2011
ISBN 978-0-7020-3127-4
Reprinted 2011 (twice)

British Library Cataloguing in Publication Data
A catalogue record for this book is available from the British Library

Library of Congress Cataloging in Publication Data
A catalog record for this book is available from the Library of Congress

Notices
Knowledge and best practice in this field are constantly changing. As new research and experience broaden our understanding, changes in research methods, professional practices, or medical treatment may become necessary.

Practitioners and researchers must always rely on their own experience and knowledge in evaluating and using any information, methods, compounds, or experiments described herein. In using such information or methods they should be mindful of their own safety and the safety of others, including parties for whom they have a professional responsibility.

With respect to any drug or pharmaceutical products identified, readers are advised to check the most current information provided (i) on procedures featured or (ii) by the manufacturer of each product to be administered, to verify the recommended dose or formula, the method and duration of administration, and contraindications. It is the responsibility of practitioners, relying on their own experience and knowledge of their patients, to make diagnoses, to determine dosages and the best treatment for each individual patient, and to take all appropriate safety precautions.

To the fullest extent of the law, neither the Publisher nor the authors, contributors, or editors, assume any liability for any injury and/or damage to persons or property as a matter of products liability, negligence or otherwise, or from any use or operation of any methods, products, instructions, or ideas contained in the material herein.

Resources that accompany this text

The chapters and appendix that comprise this book constitute a traditional way of presenting our ideas about EBM. We wanted to keep the book pocket-sized and therefore our discussion is restricted by the limits of print space. To overcome this limitation, we've provided additional materials on the accompanying CD, including resources for practicing EBM that can be downloaded to your PDA. The CD also contains clinical examples, critical appraisals and background papers from other healthcare disciplines, including nursing and occupational therapy and links to various evidence resources.

Because some of the examples used in this book will be out of date by the time you're reading this, the supporting website (www.cebm.utoronto.ca) for this book will provide updates and new materials, so we'd suggest you check it periodically. It will also be a means of contacting the authors and letting us know where we've gone wrong and what we could do better in the future.

Minimum system requirements

Windows®

Windows XP or higher
1.6 GHz or faster CPU
1 GB RAM
8× or faster CD-ROM drive
VGA monitor supporting 1024 × 768 at millions of colors
Sound Card and speakers

Macintosh®

Apple G4 1.25 GHz or faster CPU
Mac OS 10.1 or later
1 GB RAM
8× or faster CD-ROM drive
VGA monitor supporting 1024 × 768 at millions of colors

Installation instructions

Windows®

If your system does not support Autorun, navigate to your CD drive and double click on 'Start.exe' to begin.
Alternatively, click Start, Run and type 'D:Start' to begin. If D: is not your CD drive, substitute D: with the appropriate drive letter.

Macintosh®

Open the CD icon that appears on the desktop and select 'Start' to begin.

Getting Help

If you have questions or problems with the installation or use of this CD please contact technical support:
Via phone: Monday – Friday, 5:30 a.m. – 7:00 p.m. CST
Inside US and Canada Call 1-800-692-9010
Inside the United Kingdom, call 0-0800-6929-0100
Rest of World, call +1-314-872-8370
Via fax: Fax question or problem to 1-314-579-3316
Email: Send email to technical.support@elsevier.com

Please help us solve your problem by having the following information available when you contact technical support:
- Type and speed of processor (e.g. Pentium 1.6 GHz)
- Amount of RAM (e.g. 1 GB)
- Video display settings (e.g. 800 × 600, 16-bit)
- Speed of CD-ROM drive (e.g. 8×)
- Size and free space of hard disk (e.g. 80 GB total, 5 GB free)
- Operating system including version and service packs (e.g. Windows XP, service pack 2)
- Version number of the browser, available from the help pull-down menu, under About (IE or Safari)

For more information regarding other products, visit our website at www.elsevierhealth.com.

Contents

1
2
3
4
5
6
7
8
9

Contents of the CD

A. Evidence-based Medicine: how to practice and teach it

B. Bibliography of Evidence-based Health Care Resources

C. EBM Toolbox

- GATE critical appraisal worksheets
- Educational prescription
- CATMaker
- Pocket cards
- CEBM Appraisal worksheets

D. PDA tools

- EBM calculator
- NNT/LR tables
- Pocket cards
- Educational Prescription
- CQ log

Preface

This book is for clinicians at any stage of their training or career who want to learn how to practice and teach evidence-based medicine. It's been written for the busy clinician and thus, it's short and practical. The book emphasizes direct clinical application of EBM and tactics to practice and teach EBM in real-time. Those who want, and have time for, more detailed discussions of the theoretical and methodological bases for the tactics described here should consult one of the longer textbooks on clinical epidemiology.*

The focus of the book has changed with the continuing clinical experiences of the authors. For Sharon Straus the ideas behind the ongoing development of the book have built on her experiences as a medical student on a general medicine ward, when she was challenged by a senior resident to provide evidence to support her management plans for each patient she admitted. This was so much more exciting than some previous rotations, where the management plan was learned by rote and was based on whatever the current consultant favored. After residency, she undertook postgraduate training in clinical epidemiology and this further stimulated her interest in EBM, leading to a fellowship with Dave Sackett in Oxford, where her enthusiasm for practicing and teaching EBM continued to grow. She continues to learn from colleagues, mentors and trainees, stealing many of their teaching tips! She hopes that this has led to improved patient care and to more fun and challenge for her students and residents, from whom she's learned so much.

For Paul Glasziou, the first inkling of another way began when, as a newly qualified and puzzled doctor, he was fortunate enough to stumble on a copy of Henrik Wulff's *Rational Diagnosis and Treatment*. After a long journey of exploration (thanks Arthur, Jorgen, John and Les), a serendipitous visit from Dave Sackett to Sydney in the late 1980s led him to return to clinical work. A brief visit to McMaster University with Dave Sackett convinced him that research really could be used to improve

---

*We suggest: Haynes RB, Sackett DL, Guyatt GH, Tugwell P. Clinical epidemiology: How to do clinical practice research. Philadelphia: Lippincott Williams & Wilkins, 2006.

care. Feeling better armed to recognize and manage the uncertainties inherent in clinical consultations, he continues to enjoy general practice, and teaching others to record and answer their own clinical questions. He remains awed by the vast unexplored tracts of clinical practice not visible from the eyepiece of a microscope. Rather than write "what I never learnt at medical school", he is delighted to contribute to this book.

For Scott Richardson, the ideas for this book began coming together very slowly. As a beginning clinical clerk in the 1970s, one of his teachers told him to read the literature to decide what to do for his patients, but then said "of course, nobody really does that!" During residency Scott tried harder to use the literature but found few tools to help him do it effectively. Some of the ideas for this book took shape for Scott when he came across the notions of clinical epidemiology and critical appraisal in the late 1970s and early 1980s and he began to use them in his practice and teaching of students and postgraduates at the University of Rochester. On his journeys in Rochester, Hamilton, Oxford, San Antonio, Dayton, and Athens, Scott has worked with others in evidence-based medicine (including these co-authors), fashioning those earlier ideas into clinician-friendly tools for everyday use. Scott continues to have big fun learning from and teaching with a large number of EBM colleagues around the world, all working to improve the care of patients by making wise use of research evidence.

Brian Haynes started worrying about the relationship between evidence and clinical practice during his second year of medical school when a psychiatrist gave a lecture on Freud's theories. When asked, "What's the evidence that Freud's theories were correct?", the psychiatrist admitted that there wasn't any good evidence, and that he didn't believe the theories, but he had been asked by the head of the department "to give the talk". This eventually led him to a career combining clinical practice (in internal medicine) with research (in clinical epidemiology) to "get the evidence" – only to find that the evidence being generated by medical researchers around the world wasn't getting to practitioners and patients in a timely and dependable way. Sabbaticals permitted a career shift into medical informatics to look into how knowledge is disseminated and applied, and how practitioners and patients can use and benefit from "current best evidence". This led to the development of several evidence-based information resources including *ACP Journal Club*, *Evidence-Based Medicine*, *Evidence-Based Nursing*, *Evidence-Based Mental Health*, in print and electronic versions, to make it easier for practitioners to get at the best current evidence. At present, he is devising even more devious ways to get evidence into practice including making highly refined evidence so inexpensive and available that less refined evidence won't stand a chance in competing for practitioners' reading materials, computers or brains. They also say that he's a dreamer …

A note about our choice of words: we'll talk about "our" patients throughout this book, not to imply any possession or control of them by us, but to signify that we have taken on an obligation and responsibility to care for and serve each of them.

We're sure that this book contains several errors – we just don't know (yet!) what and where they are. When you find them, please go to our website and tell us about them. In return, we'll credit you in subsequent printings of the book.

For the contents of this book to benefit patients, we believe that clinicians must have a mastery of the clinical skills including history-taking, and physical examination, without which we can neither begin the process of EBM (by generating diagnostic hypotheses) nor end it (by integrating valid, important evidence with our patient's values and expectations). We also advocate continuous, self-directed, lifelong learning. As TH White wrote in *The Once and Future King*, "learning is the only thing which the mind can never exhaust, never alienate, never be tortured by, never fear or distrust, and never dream of regretting". By not regarding knowledge with humility and by denying our uncertainty and curiosity, we risk becoming dangerously out of date and immune to self-improvement and advances in medicine. Finally, we invite you to add the enthusiasm and irreverence to the endeavor without which you will miss the fun that accompanies the application of these ideas!

Acknowledgments

If this book is found to be useful, much of the credit for it is due to Muir Gray and David L. Sackett who created and led respectively, the NHS R&D Centre for Evidence-based Practice at Oxford which provided a home and working retreat for all of the authors at various times. They have provided the authors with great mentorship, and advice including, "if you can dream it, you can do it". And we thank them for encouraging us to dream, and for helping us to achieve many of those dreams.

We thank our colleagues for their infinite patience and our families for their loving support. Sharon Straus gives special thanks to Jeremy Grimshaw, Rod Jackson, Andreas Laupacis, and Art Slutsky for their mentorship; to all the students, fellows and residents for their inspiration and fun; and to Dave Sackett for his friendship and mentorship. Paul Glasziou thanks Arthur Elstein, Jorgen Hilden, John Simes, Les Irwig and Dave Sackett for their mentorship and friendship. Scott Richardson gives special thanks to Sherry Parmer and Alexandra Richardson, and to his many teachers and colleagues who have taught by example and who have given him so generously both intellectual challenge and personal support. Brian Haynes thanks the American College of Physicians and the BMJ Publishing Group for leading the way in providing opportunities to create and disseminate many of the "evidence-based" information resources featured in this book and its companion CD and website.

We're still seeking better ways of explaining these ideas and their clinical application, and will acknowledge readers' suggestions in subsequent editions of this book. In the meantime, we take cheerful responsibility for the parts of the current edition that are still fuzzy, wrong, or boring.

Introduction

What is EBM?

Evidence-based medicine (EBM) requires the integration of the best research evidence with our clinical expertise and our patient's unique values and circumstances.

- By *best research evidence* we mean clinically relevant research, sometimes from the basic sciences of medicine, but especially from patient-centered clinical research into the accuracy and precision of diagnostic tests (including the clinical examination), the power of prognostic markers, and the efficacy and safety of therapeutic, rehabilitative, and preventive strategies.

- By *clinical expertise* we mean the ability to use our clinical skills and past experience to rapidly identify each patient's unique health state and diagnosis, their individual risks and benefits of potential interventions, and their personal values and expectations.

- By *patient values* we mean the unique preferences, concerns and expectations each patient brings to a clinical encounter and which must be integrated into clinical decisions if they are to serve the patient.

- By *patient circumstances* we mean their individual clinical state and the clinical setting.

Why the interest in EBM?

Interest in EBM has grown exponentially since the coining of the term[1] in 1992 by a group led by Gordon Guyatt at McMaster University, from one MEDLINE citation in 1992 to over 57 000 in October 2009. Searching Google and Google Scholar with the terms evidence-based medicine retrieves almost 10 million hits and more than 2.5 million hits, respectively. Moreover, evidence-based practice has become incorporated into many healthcare disciplines including occupational therapy, physiotherapy, nursing, dentistry, and complementary medicine among many others. Indeed, we've been told by one publisher that adding evidence-based to the title of a book can increase sales – regardless of whether the book is evidence-based! Professional organizations and training programs for various healthcare professionals have moved from whether to teach EBM to how to teach it, resulting in an explosion in the number of courses, workshops and seminars offered in this practice. Similarly, EBM educational interventions for the public, policy-makers and healthcare managers have grown.

The spread of EBM has arisen from several realizations:

1. Our daily need for valid and quantitative information about diagnosis, prognosis, therapy and prevention (up to five times per inpatient[2] and twice for every three outpatients[3]).

2. The inadequacy of traditional sources for this information because they are out of date (traditional textbooks[4]), frequently wrong (experts[5]), ineffective (didactic continuing medical education[6]) or too overwhelming in their volume and too variable in their validity for practical clinical use (medical journals[7]).

3. The disparity between our diagnostic skills and clinical judgment, which increase with experience, and our up-to-date knowledge[8] and clinical performance[9] which decline.

4. Our inability to afford more than a few seconds per patient for finding and assimilating this evidence[10] or to set aside more than half an hour per week for general reading and study.[11]

5. The gaps between evidence and practice (including overuse and underuse of evidence) lead to variations in practice and quality of care.[12-14]

These challenges have been met with a number of potential solutions which facilitate the practice of EBM:

1. The development of strategies for efficiently tracking down and appraising evidence (for its validity and relevance).

2. The creation of evidence synopsis and summary services which allow us to find and use high-quality pre-appraised evidence.[15]

3. The creation of information systems for bringing these evidence resources to us within seconds.[10]

4. The identification and application of effective strategies for lifelong learning and for improving our clinical performance.[16]

This book is devoted to describing these innovations, demonstrating their application to clinical problems, and showing how they can be learned and practiced by clinicians who have just 30 minutes per week to devote to their continuing professional development.

How do we practice EBM?

The complete practice of EBM comprises five steps, and this book addresses each in turn:

- *Step 1:* converting the need for information (about prevention, diagnosis, prognosis, therapy, causation, etc.) into an answerable question (Ch. 1).
- *Step 2:* tracking down the best evidence with which to answer that question (Ch. 2).
- *Step 3:* critically appraising that evidence for its validity (closeness to the truth), impact (size of the effect), and applicability (usefulness in our clinical practice) (the first halves of Chs 3–7).
- *Step 4:* integrating the critical appraisal with our clinical expertise and with our patient's unique biology, values and circumstances (the second halves of Chs 3–7).
- *Step 5:* evaluating our effectiveness and efficiency in executing steps 1–4 and seeking ways to improve them both for next time (Ch. 8).

When we examine our practice and that of our colleagues and trainees in this five-step fashion, we identify that clinicians can incorporate evidence into their practices in three ways. First, is the "doing" mode, in which at least the first four steps above are completed. Second, is the "using" mode in which searches are restricted to evidence resources that have already undergone critical appraisal by others, such as evidence summaries (thus skipping Step 3). Third, is the "replicating" mode in which the decisions of respected opinion leaders are followed (abandoning at least Steps 2 and 3). All three of these modes involve the integration of evidence (from whatever source) with our patient's unique biology, values and circumstances of Step 4, but they vary in the execution of the other steps. For the conditions we encounter every day (e.g. acute coronary syndrome and venous thromboembolism), we need to be "up to the minute" and very sure about what we are doing. Accordingly, we invest the time and effort necessary to carry out both Steps 2 (searching) and 3 (critically appraising), and operate in the "doing" mode; all the chapters in this book are relevant to this mode. For the conditions we encounter less often (e.g. salicylate overdose), we conserve our time by seeking out critical appraisals already performed by others who describe (and stick to!) explicit criteria for deciding what evidence they selected and how they decided whether it was valid. We omit the time-consuming Step 3 (critically appraising) and carry out just Step 2 (searching) but restrict the latter to sources that have already undergone rigorous critical appraisal (e.g. *ACP Journal Club*). Only the third portions ("Can I apply this valid, important evidence to my patient?") of Chapters 3–7 are strictly relevant here, and the growing database of pre-appraised resources (described in Ch. 2) is making this "using" mode more and more feasible for busy clinicians. For the problems we're likely to encounter very infrequently (e.g., graft vs host disease in a bone marrow transplant recipient), we "blindly" seek, accept and apply the recommendations we receive from authorities in the relevant branch of medicine. This "replicating" mode also characterizes the practice of medical students and clinical trainees when they haven't yet been granted independence and have to carry out the orders of their consultants. The trouble with the "replicating" mode is that it is "blind" to whether the advice received from the experts is authoritative (evidence-based, resulting from their operating in the "appraising" mode) or merely authoritarian (opinion-based). Sometimes we can gain clues about the validity of our expert source (e.g., do they cite references?). If we tracked the care we give when operating in the "replicating" mode into the literature and critically appraised it, we would find that some of it was effective, some useless, and some harmful. But in the "replicating" mode we'll never be sure which.

The authors of this book don't practice as EBM doers all of the time and we find that we move between the different modes of practicing EBM depending on the clinical scenario, the frequency with which it arises, and the time and resources available to address our clinical questions. And, while some clinicians may want to become proficient in practicing all five steps of EBM, many others would instead prefer to focus on becoming efficient users (and knowledge managers) of evidence. This book tries to meet the needs of these various end-users. And, for those readers who are teachers of EBM, we try to describe various ways in which the learning needs of the different learners can be achieved, including those who want to be primarily users or doers of EBM.

Can clinicians practice EBM?

Surveys conducted among clinicians from various disciplines have found that clinicians are interested in learning the necessary skills for practicing EBM.[17,18] One survey of the UK GPs suggests that many clinicians already practice in the "using" mode, using evidence-based summaries generated by others (72%) and evidence-based practice guidelines or protocols (84%).[18] Far fewer claimed to understand (and to be able to explain) the "appraising" tools of NNTs (35%) and confidence intervals (CIs) (20%). Several studies have found that participants' understandings of EBM concepts are quite variable.[19,20]

If clinicians have the necessary skills for practicing EBM, can it be done in real-time? When a busy (180+ admissions per month) inpatient medical service brought electronic summaries of evidence previously appraised either by team members ("CATS") or by synopsis resources to working rounds, it was documented that, on average, the former could be accessed in 10 seconds and the latter in 25.[10] Moreover, when assessed from the viewpoint of the most junior members of the team caring for the patient, this evidence changed 25% of their diagnostic and treatment suggestions and added to a further 23% of them. This study has been replicated in other clinical settings, including an obstetrical service.[21] Finally, clinical audits from many practice settings have found that there is a significant evidence base for the primary interventions that are encountered on these clinical services.[22–29]

What's the "E" for EBM?

There is an accumulating body of evidence relating to the impact of EBM on healthcare professionals from systematic reviews of training in the skills of EBM[30] to qualitative research describing the experience of EBM practitioners.[31] Indeed, since the last edition of this book was published, there has been an explosion in the number of studies evaluating EBM educational interventions targeting undergraduates, postgraduates and practicing clinicians. However, these studies of the effect of teaching and practicing EBM are challenging to conduct. In many studies, the intervention has been difficult to define. It's unclear what the appropriate "dose" or "formulation" should be. Some studies use an approach to clinical practice while others use training in one of the discrete "microskills" of EBM such as MEDLINE searching[32] or critical appraisal.[33] Studies have evaluated online, in-person, small-group and large-group educational interventions.[34] Learners have different learning needs and styles and these differences must be reflected in the educational experiences provided.

Just as the intervention has proved difficult to define, the evaluation of whether the intervention has met its goals has been challenging. Effective EBM interventions will produce a wide range of outcomes. Changes in knowledge and skills are relatively easy to detect and demonstrate. Changes in attitudes and behaviors are harder to confirm. Randomized studies of EBM educational interventions have shown that these interventions can change knowledge and attitudes.[35] Similarly randomized trials have shown that these interventions can enhance EBM skills.[34,36] A study has shown that a multi-faceted EBM educational intervention (including access to evidence resources and a seminar series using real clinical scenarios) significantly improved evidence-based practice patterns in a district general hospital.[37] Still more challenging is detecting changes in clinical outcomes. Studies of undergraduate and postgraduate educational interventions have shown limited impact on ongoing behavior or clinical outcomes.[34,38] Studies demonstrating better patient survival when practice is evidence-based (and worse when it isn't) are limited to outcomes research.[39,40] We are still waiting to see a trial where access to evidence is withheld from control clinicians.

Along with the interest in EBM, interest in evaluating EBM and developing evaluation instruments has grown. There are several instruments available for evaluating EBM educational interventions including those that assess attitudes, knowledge and skills. We encourage interested readers to review the recent systematic review which addresses this topic.[41] For any educational intervention, we encourage teachers and researchers to consider that it is necessary to consider changes in performance and outcomes over time because EBM requires lifelong learning and this is not something that can be measured over the short term.

By questioning the "E" for EBM, are we asking the right question? It has been recognized that providing evidence from clinical research is a necessary but not sufficient condition for the provision of optimal care. This has created interest in knowledge translation, the scientific study of the methods for closing the knowledge-to-practice gap and the analysis of barriers and facilitators inherent in this process.[42] Proponents of knowledge translation have identified that changing behavior is a complex process requiring comprehensive approaches directed towards patients, physicians, managers and policy-makers and provision of evidence is but one component. In this edition, we'll touch briefly on knowledge translation which focuses on evidence-based implementation. This is not the primary focus of the book which instead targets the practice of individual clinicians, patients and teachers.

What are the limitations of EBM?

Discussion about the practice of EBM naturally engenders negative and positive reactions from clinicians. Some of the criticisms focus on misunderstandings and misperceptions of EBM such as the concerns that it ignores patient values and preferences and promotes a cookbook approach (for interested readers, we refer you to a systematic review of the criticisms of EBM and to a more recent editorial discussing these).[43,44] An examination of the definition and steps of EBM quickly dismisses these criticisms. Evidence, whether strong or weak, is never sufficient to make clinical decisions. Individual values and preferences must balance this evidence to achieve optimal shared decision-making and highlight that the practice of EBM is not a "one-size fits all" approach. Other critics have expressed worry that EBM will be hijacked by managers to promote cost-cutting. However, it is not an effective cost-cutting tool, since providing evidence-based care directed toward maximizing patients' quality of life often increases the costs of their care and raises the ire of some health economists.[45] The self-reported employment of the "using" mode by a great majority of front-line GPs dispels the contention that EBM is an ivory tower concept, another common criticism. Finally, we hope that the rest of this book will put to rest the concern that EBM leads to therapeutic nihilism in the absence of randomized trial evidence. Proponents of EBM would acknowledge that several sources of evidence inform clinical decision-making. The practice of EBM stresses finding the best available evidence to answer a question, and this evidence may come from randomized trials, rigorous observational studies, or even anecdotal reports from experts. Hierarchies of evidence have been developed to help describe the quality of evidence that may be found to answer clinical questions. Randomized trials and systematic reviews of randomized trials provide the highest quality evidence – that is, the lowest likelihood of bias, and thus the lowest likelihood to mislead because they establish the effect of an intervention. However, they are not usually the best sources for answering questions about diagnosis, prognosis, or the harmful impact of potentially noxious exposures.

This debate has highlighted limitations unique to the practice of EBM that must be considered. For example, the need to develop new skills in seeking and appraising evidence cannot be underestimated. And, the need to develop and apply these skills within the time constraints of our clinical practice must be addressed.

This book attempts to tackle these limitations and offers potential solutions. For example, EBM skills can be acquired at any stage in clinical training and members of clinical teams at various stages of training can collaborate by sharing the searching and appraising tasks. Incorporating the acquisition of these skills into grand rounds, as well as postgraduate and undergraduate seminars integrates them with the other skills being developed in these settings. These strategies are discussed at length in Chapter 8. Important developments to help overcome the limited time and resources include the growing numbers of evidence-based journals and evidence-based summary services. These are discussed throughout the book and in detail in Chapter 2. Indeed, one of the goals of this edition of the book is to provide tips and tools for practicing EBM in "real-time". And, we encourage readers to use the website to let us know about ways in which they've managed to meet the challenges of practicing EBM in real-time. (For learners and teachers who encounter criticisms of EBM, we've included a presentation on the accompanying CD which outlines the limitations of EBM and potential solutions).

How is this package (the book, the accompanying CD, and the associated website) organized?

The overall package is designed to help practitioners from any healthcare discipline learn how to practice evidence-based healthcare. Thus, although the book is written within the perspectives of internal medicine and general practice, the CD provides clinical scenarios, questions, searches, critical appraisals, and evidence summaries from other disciplines, permitting readers to apply the strategies and tactics of evidence-based practice to any health discipline.

For those of you who want to become more proficient "doers" of EBM, we suggest that you take a look at Chapters 1 through 9. For readers who want to become "users" of EBM, we suggest tackling Chapters 1 and 2, focusing on question formulation and matching those questions to the various evidence resources. We have also provided tips on practicing EBM in real-time throughout the book and on the accompanying CD. Finally, for those interested in teaching the practice of EBM, we have dedicated Chapter 8 to this topic.

The chapters and appendix that comprise this book constitute a traditional way of presenting our ideas about EBM. It offers the "basic" (or "Ka") version of the model for practicing EBM. For those who want more detailed discussion, we suggest you review some other resources.[46] And, while the examples were current when we wrote this in 2010, by the time this book appears in print, they may be outdated! So, we suggest that you visit our website for ongoing materials and practice tools (www.cebm.utoronto.ca). This website can also be used to contact us; in particular, we'd like to hear where we've gone wrong and what we could do better in future editions.

References

1. Evidence-based Medicine Working Group. Evidence-based medicine. A new approach to teaching the practice of medicine. *JAMA*. 1992;268:2420–2425.

2. Osheroff JA, Forsythe DE, Buchanan BG, et al. Physicians' information needs: analysis of questions posed during clinical teaching. *Ann Intern Med*. 1991;114:576–581.

3. Covell DG, Uman GC, Manning PR. Information needs in office practice: are they being met? *Ann Intern Med*. 1985;103:596–599.

4. Antman EM, Lau J, Kupelnick B, et al. A comparison of results of meta-analyses of randomised control trials and recommendations of clinical experts. *JAMA*. 1992;268:240–248.

5. Oxman A, Guyatt GH. The science of reviewing research. *Ann N Y Acad Sci*. 1993;703:125–134.

6. Davis D, O'Brien MA, Freemantle N, et al. Impact of formal continuing medical education. *JAMA*. 1999;282:867–874.

7. Haynes RB. Where's the meat in clinical journals [editorial]? *ACP J Club*. 1993;119:A-22–A-23.

8. Evans CE, Haynes RB, Birkett NJ, et al. Does a mailed continuing education program improve clinician performance? Results of a randomised trial in antihypertensive care. *JAMA*. 1986;255:501–504.

9. Sackett DL, Haynes RB, Taylor DW, et al. Clinical determinants of the decision to treat primary hypertension. *Clin Res*. 1977;24:648.

10. Sackett DL, Straus SE. Finding and applying evidence during clinical rounds: the 'evidence cart'. *JAMA*. 1998;280:1336–1338.

11. Sackett DL. Using evidence-based medicine to help physicians keep up-to-date. *Serials*. 1997;9:178–181.

12. Shah BR, Mamdani M, Jaakkimainen L, et al. Risk modification for diabetic patients. *Can J Clin Pharmacol*. 2004;11:239–244.

13. Pimlott NJ, Hux JE, Wilson LM, et al. Educating physicians to reduce benzodiazepine use by elderly patients. *CMAJ*. 2003;168:835–839.

14. Kennedy J, Quan H, Ghali WA, et al. Variations in rates of appropriate and inappropriate carotid endarterectomy for stroke prevention in 4 Canadian provinces. *CMAJ*. 2004;171:455–459.

15. Haynes RB, Cotoi C, Holland J, et al. Second-order peer review of the medical literature for clinical practitioners. *JAMA*. 2006;295:1801–1808.

16. Effective practice and organization of care group. *The Cochrane Library*. London: Wiley; 2009.

17. McAlister FA, Graham I, Karr GW, et al. Evidence-based medicine and the practicing clinician: a survey of Canadian general internists. *JGIM*. 1999;14:236–242.

18. McColl A, Smith H, White P, et al. General practitioners' perceptions of the route to evidence-based medicine: a questionnaire survey. *BMJ*. 1998;316:361–365.

19. Young JM, Glasziou P, Ward J. General practitioners' self ratings of skills in evidence based medicine: validation study. *BMJ*. 2002;324:950–951.

20. Sekimoto M, Imanaka Y, Kitano N, et al. Why are physicians not persuaded by scientific evidence? *BMC Health Serv Res*. 2006;6:92.

21. Deshpande N, Publicover M, Gee H, et al. Incorporating the views of obstetric clinicians in implementing evidence-supported labor and delivery suite ward rounds: a case study. *Health Info Libr J*. 2003;20(2):86–94.

22. Ellis J, Mulligan I, Rowe J, et al. In-patient general medicine is evidence based. *Lancet*. 1995;346:407–410.

23. Geddes JR, Game D, Jenkins NE, et al. In-patient psychiatric care is evidence-based. In: *Proceedings of the Royal College of Psychiatrists Winter Meeting*, Stratford, UK, January 1996:23–25.

24. Howes N, Chagla L, Thorpe M, et al. Surgical practice is evidence based. *Br J Surg*. 1997;84:1220–1223.

25. Kenny SE, Shankar KR, Rintala R, et al. Evidence-based surgery: interventions in a regional paediatric surgical unit. *Arch Dis Child*. 1997;76:50–53.

26. Gill P, Dowell AC, Neal RD, et al. Evidence based general practice: a retrospective study of interventions in one training practice. *BMJ*. 1996;312:819–821.

27. Moyer VA, Gist AK, Elliott EJ. Is the practice of pediatric in-patient medicine evidence-based? *J Pediatr Child Health*. 2002;38:347–351.

28. Waters KL, Wiebe N, Cramer K, et al. Treatment in the pediatric emergency department is evidence based: a retrospective analysis. *BMC Pediatr*. 2006;6:26.

29. Lai TY, Wong VW, Leung GM. Is ophthalmology evidence based? *Br J Ophthalmol*. 2003;87:385–390.

30. Parkes J, Hyde C, Deeks J, et al. Teaching critical appraisal skills in health care settings. *Cochrane Database of Syst Rev*. 2001;(3): CD001270.

31. Greenhalgh T, Douglas HR. Experiences of general practitioners and practice nurses of training courses in evidence-based health care: a qualitative study. *Br J Gen Pract*. 1999;49:536–540.

32. Rosenberg W, Deeks J, Lusher A, et al. Improving searching skills and evidence retrieval. *J Roy Coll Phys*. 1998;328:557–563.

33. Taylor RS, Reeves BC, Ewings PE, et al. Critical appraisal skills training for health care professionals: a randomised controlled trial. *BMD Med Educ*. 2004;4:30.

34. Bradley P, Oterhold C, Herrin J, et al. Comparison of directed and self-directed learning in evidence-based medicine: a randomised controlled trial. *Med Educ*. 2005;39:1027–1035.

35. Johnston J, Schooling CM, Leung GM. A randomised controlled trial of two educational modes for undergraduate evidence-based medicine learning in Asia. *BMC Med Educ*. 2009;9:63.

36. Shnval K, Berkovits E, Netzer D, et al. Evaluating the impact of an evidence-based medicine educational intervention on primary care doctors' attitudes, knowledge and clinical behavior: a controlled trial and before and after study. *J Eval Clin Pract*. 2007;13:581–598.

37. Straus SE, Ball C, Balcombe N, et al. Teaching evidence-based medicine skills can change practice in a community hospital. *JGIM*. 2005;20(4):340–343.

38. Kim S, Willett LR, Murphy DJ, et al. Impact of an evidence-based medicine curriculum on resident use of electronic resources. *JGIM*. 2008;23:1804–1808.

39. Mitchell JB, Ballard DJ, Whisnant JP, et al. What role do neurologists play in determining the costs and outcomes of stroke patients? *Stroke*. 1996;27:1937–1943.

40. Wong JH, Findlay JM, Suarez-Almazor ME. Regional performance of carotid endarterectomy appropriateness, outcomes and risk factors for complications. *Stroke*. 1997;28:891–898.

41. Shaneyfelt T, Baum KD, Bell D, et al. Instruments for evaluating education in evidence-based practice. *JAMA*. 2006;296:1116–1127.

42. Straus SE, Tetroe J, Graham ID. Defining knowledge translation. *CMAJ*. 2009;181:165–168.

43. Straus SE, McAlister FA. Evidence-based medicine: a commentary on common criticisms. *CMAJ*. 2000;163:837–841.

44. Straus SE, Glasziou P, Haynes RB, et al. Misunderstandings, misperceptions and mistakes. *ACP JC*. 2007;146:A8.

45. Maynard A. Evidence-based medicine: an incomplete method for informing treatment choices. *Lancet*. 1997;349:126–128.

46. Guyatt G, Rennie D, Meade M, et al., eds. *Users' guides to the medical literature. A manual for evidence-based clinical practice*. Chicago: AMA press; 2008.

1 Asking answerable clinical questions

As noted in the Introduction, as we care for patients we will often need new healthcare knowledge to inform our decisions and actions.[1-3] Our learning needs can involve several types of useful knowledge, and can range from simple, and readily available to complex, subtle, and much harder to find. In this chapter we describe strategies for the first step in meeting these knowledge needs: asking clinical questions that are answerable with evidence from clinical care research. We will start with a patient encounter to remind us how clinical questions arise and to show how they can be used to initiate evidence-based clinical learning. We will also introduce some teaching tactics that can help us coach others to develop their questioning skills.

Clinical scenario

You've just begun a month as the attending physician supervising residents and students on a hospital medicine inpatient service. You join the team on rounds after they've finished admitting a patient. The patient is an 81-year-old woman admitted with a history of progressive dyspnea, leg edema and pallor over the last 3 months. She had previously been healthy, with no chronic conditions, on no medications, and requiring no assistance. Her exam shows striking pallor, pitting edema of both shins, diminished position and vibratory sensation over her feet and ankles, along with the absence of neck vein distension or an S3 gallop. Her chest radiograph is normal. Test results include a very low hemoglobin, an increased mean corpuscular volume, and a very low blood level of vitamin B12.

You ask your team for their questions about important pieces of medical knowledge they'd like to have in order to provide better care for this patient. What do you expect they would ask? What questions occur to you about this patient? Write the first three of your questions in the boxes below:

> 1.

> 2.

> 3.

The team's medical students asked several questions, including these three:

a. What are the causes of vitamin B12 deficiency?

b. How does B12 deficiency lead to loss of vibratory and position sensation?

c. How long does B12 deficiency take to develop from lack of the vitamin in the diet?

The team's house officers also asked several questions, including these three:

a. Among patients found to have vitamin B12 deficiency who undergo a thorough evaluation, how frequently would each of the important underlying disease categories be diagnosed?

b. In adults with severe anemia from B12 deficiency, would chronic oral B12 supplementation (after initial parenteral repletion) yield similar symptomatic and hematologic response as chronic parenteral supplementation, with lower cost and fewer adverse effects?

c. In patients with some loss of position and vibratory sensation present at the time of the diagnosis of vitamin B12 deficiency, how likely are these neurologic findings to disappear, stay the same, or progressively worsen despite treatment over the next months and years?

Background and foreground questions

Note that the students' questions concern general knowledge that would help them understand B12 deficiency as a disorder. Such "background" questions can be asked about any disorder or health state, a test, a treatment or intervention, or other aspect of healthcare, and can encompass biologic, psychologic, or sociologic phenomena.[4] When well formulated, such background questions usually have two components (Table 1.1):

1. A question root (who, what, when, where, how, why) with a verb.

2. An aspect of the condition or thing of interest.

Note that the house officers' questions concern specific knowledge that could directly inform one or more "foreground" clinical decisions they face with this patient, including a broad range of biologic, psychologic, and sociologic issues. When well built, such foreground questions usually have four components (Table 1.1)[5,6]:

1. The *patient* situation, *population*, or problem of interest.

2. The main *intervention*, defined very broadly, including an exposure, a diagnostic test, a prognostic factor, a treatment, a patient perception, and so forth.

Table 1.1 Well-built clinical questions

"Background" questions

- Ask for general knowledge about a condition, test, or treatment
- Have two essential components:
  1. A question root (who, what, where, when, how, why) and a verb
  2. A disorder, test, treatment, or other aspect of healthcare

Examples:
"How does heart failure cause pleural effusions?"
"What causes swine flu?"

"Foreground" questions

- Ask for specific knowledge to inform clinical decisions or actions
- Have 4 essential components:
  1. "P": Patient, population, predicament, or problem
  2. "I": Intervention, exposure, test, or other agent
  3. "C": Comparison intervention, exposure, test, etc., if relevant
  4. "O": Outcomes of clinical importance, including time when relevant

Example:
"In adults with heart failure with reduced systolic function, would adding the implantation of an electronic resynchronization device to standard therapy reduce morbidity or mortality enough over 3–5 years to be worth the potential additional harmful effects and costs?"

---

3. A *comparison* intervention or exposure (also defined very broadly), if relevant.

4. The clinical *outcome(s)* of interest, including a time horizon, if relevant.

Return to the three questions you wrote down about this patient. Are they background or foreground questions? Do your background questions specify two components (root with verb and condition), and do your foreground questions contain three or four components (patient/problem, intervention, comparison, and outcomes)? If not, try rewriting them to include these components, and consider whether these revised questions come closer to asking what you really want to know.

As clinicians, we all have needs for both background and foreground knowledge, in proportions that vary over time and that depend primarily on our experience with the particular disorder at hand (Figure 1.1). When our experience with the condition is limited, at point "A" (like a beginning student), the majority of our questions (shown in Figure 1.1 by the vertical dimension) might be about background knowledge. As we grow in clinical experience and responsibility, such as point "B" (like a house officer), we'll have increasing proportions of questions about the foreground of managing patients. Further experience with the condition puts us at point "C" (like a consultant), where most of our questions will be foreground. Notice the diagonal line is placed to show that we're never too green to learn foreground knowledge, nor too experienced to outlive the need for background knowledge.

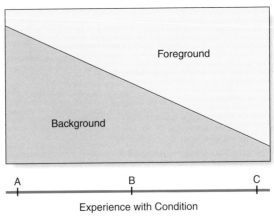

Figure 1.1 Knowledge needs depend on experience with condition.

Our reactions to knowing and to not knowing

Clinical practice demands that we use large amounts of both background and foreground knowledge, whether or not we're aware of their use. These demands and our awareness come in three combinations, which we'll examine here. First, our patient's predicament may call for knowledge we know we already possess, so we will experience the reinforcing mental and emotional responses termed "cognitive resonance" as we apply the knowledge in clinical decisions. Second, we may realize that our patient's illness calls for knowledge we don't possess, and this awareness brings the mental and emotional responses termed "cognitive dissonance" as we confront what we don't know, but need to know. Third, our patient's predicament might call upon knowledge we don't have, yet these gaps may escape our attention, so we don't know what we don't know and we carry on in undisturbed ignorance. (We'll return to this third situation in Chapter 2, where we'll introduce strategies to regularly strengthen and update our knowledge of current best evidence.)

Reflect for a moment on how you've learned to react to the first two situations noted above. When teachers asked questions to which you knew the answers, did you learn to raise your hand to be called upon to give the answers? We did, and so did virtually all of our learners, and in the process, we've learned that teachers and examinations reward us for already knowing the answer. When teachers asked questions to which you didn't know the answers, did you learn to raise your hand to be called upon and say "I don't know this, but I can see how useful it would be to know and I'm ready to learn it today"? Didn't think so, and neither did we, or our learners, so in the process, we've all learned that teachers and examinations do not reward us for showing our ignorance and being ready and willing to learn. And while hiding our ignorance in the classroom may have proved useful in the short run, in the long run it becomes maladaptive in clinical practice if we continue to try to hide our knowledge gaps from ourselves and avoid learning, for it will be our patients who will pay the price.

These situations of cognitive dissonance (we know that we don't know) can become powerful motivators for learning, if handled well, such as by celebrating the finding of knowledge needs and by turning the "negative space" of knowledge gaps into the "positive space" of well-built clinical questions and learning how to find the answers.[7,8] Unfortunately, if handled less well, our cognitive dissonance might lead us to less adaptive behaviors, such as trying to hide our deficits, or by reacting with anger, fear, or shame.[9] By developing awareness of our knowing and thinking, we can recognize our cognitive dissonance when it occurs, recognize when the knowledge we need will come from clinical care research, and articulate the background or foreground questions that we can use to find the answers.

Where and how clinical questions arise

Over the years, we've found that most of our foreground questions arise around the central issues involved in caring for patients (Table 1.2). These groupings are neither jointly exhaustive (other worthwhile questions can be asked), nor mutually exclusive (some questions are hybrids, asking about both prognosis and therapy, for example). Still we find it useful to anticipate that many of our questions will arise from common locations on this "map": clinical findings, etiology and risk, differential diagnosis, diagnostic tests, prognosis, therapy, prevention, patient experience and meaning, and self-improvement. We keep this list handy and use it to help locate the source of our knowledge deficits when we recognize the "stuck" feelings of our cognitive dissonance. Once we've

---

Table 1.2 Central issues in clinical work, where clinical questions often arise

1. **Clinical findings**: how to properly gather and interpret findings from the history and physical examination.
2. **Etiology/risk**: how to identify causes or risk factors for disease (including iatrogenic harms).
3. **Clinical manifestations of disease**: knowing how often and when a disease causes its clinical manifestations and how to use this knowledge in classifying our patients' illnesses.
4. **Differential diagnosis**: when considering the possible causes of our patients' clinical problems, how to select those that are likely, serious, and responsive to treatment.
5. **Diagnostic tests**: how to select and interpret diagnostic tests, in order to confirm or exclude a diagnosis, based on considering their precision, accuracy, acceptability, safety, expense, etc.
6. **Prognosis**: how to estimate our patient's likely clinical course over time and anticipate likely complications of the disorder.
7. **Therapy**: how to select treatments to offer our patients, that do more good than harm and that are worth the efforts and costs of using them.
8. **Prevention**: how to reduce the chance of disease by identifying and modifying risk factors and how to diagnose disease early by screening.
9. **Experience and meaning**: how to empathize with our patients' situations, appreciate the meaning they find in the experience, and understand how this meaning influences their healing.
10. **Improvement**: how to keep up-to-date, improve our clinical and other skills, and run a better, more efficient clinical care system.

---

recognized our knowledge gaps, articulating the questions can be done quickly, usually in 15–30 seconds.

Over the years, we've also found that many of our knowledge needs occur around, or during, our clinical encounters with patients. While often they arise first in our heads, just as often they are voiced at least in part by our patients. For instance, when our patients ask "What is the matter?" this relates to questions about diagnosis that are in our minds. Similarly, "What will this mean for me?" conjures both prognosis, and experience and meaning questions, while "What should be done?" brings up issues of treatment and prevention. No matter who initiates the questions, we count finding relevant answers as one of the ways we serve our patients, and to indicate this responsibility, we call these questions "ours". When we can manage to do so, we find it helpful to negotiate explicitly with our patients about which questions should be addressed, in what order, and by when. Increasingly, our patients want to work with us on answering some of these questions.

Practicing EBM in real-time

Since our patients' illness burdens are large, and our available time is small, we find that we usually have many more questions than time to answer them. For this, we recommend three strategies: capturing or saving, scheduling, and selecting.

First, because unsaved questions become unanswered questions, it follows that we need practical methods to rapidly capture and save questions for later retrieval and searching. Having just encouraged you to articulate your questions fully, it may surprise you that we recommend using very brief notations when recording questions on the run, using shorthand that makes sense to you. For instance, when we jot down "S3 DxT HF", we mean "Among adults presenting with dyspnea, how accurate is the clinical finding S3 gallop in confirming or excluding the diagnosis of congestive heart failure, when compared with a reference standard?" Note that while the shorthand often has the P, I, C, and O elements visible within it, it needn't always have, as long as it reminds you what your question really was.

How best to record these questions? Over the years, we've tried, or heard of others trying, several solutions:

1. Jotting brief notes on a blank A4-sized page with four columns pre-drawn, labeled "P", "I", "C", and "O", for each of the elements of foreground questions; this can be used by itself, or along with a separate sheet for questions about background knowledge.

2. Keying brief notes into a similarly-arrayed electronic file on a desktop computer.

3. Dictating spoken questions into a pocket-sized recording device.

4. Jotting concise questions onto actual prescription blanks (and trying to avoid giving them to the patient instead of their actual prescriptions!).

5. Jotting shorthand notes onto blank 3 by 5 cards kept in our pocket.

6. Turning on a personal digital assistant (PDA) and tapping in similar shorthand notes.

Whenever we've timed ourselves, we find it takes us about 15 seconds to record our questions with a PDA,[10] and about 5–10 seconds when recording on paper.

Second, by "scheduling", we mean deciding by when we need to have our questions answered, in particular considering when the resulting decisions need to be made. While integrated clinical care and information systems may improve to the point where our questions will be answerable at the time they arise, for most of us, this is not yet the case, and we need to be realistic in planning our time. With a moment of reflection, you can usually discern the few questions that demand immediate answers from the majority that can be scheduled to be answered later that day or at the next scheduled appointment.

Third, by "selecting", we mean deciding which one or few of the many questions we asked, or could have asked, should be pursued. This decision requires judgment and we'd suggest you consider the nature of the patient's illness, the nature of your knowledge needs, the specific clinical decisions in which you'll use the knowledge, and your role in that decision process. Then, try this sequence of filters:

a. Which question is most important to the patient's well-being, whether biologic, psychologic, or sociologic?

b. Which question is most relevant to your/your learners' knowledge needs?

c. Which question is most feasible to answer within the time you have available?

d. Which question is most interesting to you, your learners, or your patient?

e. Which question is most likely to recur in your practice?

With a moment of reflection on these explicit criteria, you can usually select one or two questions that best pass these tests and will best inform the decisions at hand.

In addition, some colleagues have developed software to use on PDAs that help you develop and save your questions. For example, "PICOmaker" can be saved to your Palm (www.library.ualberta.ca/pdazone/pico/), and on this book's accompanying CD, we've provided another example of one that you can try. Once installed, these software programs sit in your pocket, waiting to guide you through the steps of formulating questions and saving them for later retrieval.

Why bother formulating questions clearly?

1

Our own experiences suggest that well-formulated questions can help in seven ways:

1. They help us focus our scarce learning time on evidence that is directly relevant to our patients' clinical needs.

2. They help us focus our scarce learning time on evidence that directly addresses our particular knowledge needs, or those of our learners.

3. They can suggest high-yield search strategies (see Ch. 2).

4. They suggest the forms that useful answers might take (see Chs 3–7).

5. When sending or receiving a patient in referral, they can help us to communicate more clearly with our colleagues.

6. When teaching, they can help our learners to better understand the content of what we teach, while also modeling some adaptive processes for lifelong learning.

7. When our questions get answered, our knowledge grows, our curiosity is reinforced, our cognitive resonance is restored, and we can become better, faster, and happier clinicians.

In addition, the research we've seen so far suggests that clinicians who are taught this structured approach ask more specific questions,[11] undertake more searches for evidence,[12] use more detailed search methods and find more precise answers.[13,14] Also, when family doctors include a clinical question that is clearly articulated when they "curbside consult" their specialty colleagues, they are more likely to receive an answer.[15] Some groups have begun to implement and evaluate question–answer services for their clinicians, with similarly promising initial results.[16,17] A randomized trial of one such service found that providing timely answers to clinical questions had a highly positive impact on decision-making.[18]

Teaching the asking of answerable clinical questions

Good questions are the backbone of both practicing and teaching EBM, and patients serve as the starting point for both. Our challenge as teachers is to identify questions that are both patient-based (arising out of the clinical problems of this real patient under the learner's care) and learner-centered (targeting the learning needs of this learner). As we become more skilled at asking questions ourselves, we should also become more skilled in teaching others how to do so.

As with other clinical or learning skills, we can teach question-asking powerfully by role-modeling the formation of good questions in front of our learners. Doing this also lets us model admission that we don't know it all, identifying our own knowledge gaps, and showing our learners adaptive ways of responding to the resulting cognitive dissonance. Once we've modeled asking a few questions, we can stop and describe explicitly what we did, noting each of the elements of good questions, whether background or foreground.

The four main steps in teaching clinical learners how to ask good questions are listed in Table 1.3. If we are to recognize potential questions in learners' cases, help them select the "best" question to focus on, guide them in building that question well, and assess their question-building performance and skill, we need to be proficient at building questions ourselves. Moreover, we need several general attributes of good teaching, such as good listening skills, enthusiasm, and a willingness to help learners develop to their full potential. It also helps to be able to spot signs of our learners' cognitive dissonance, to know when and what they're ready to learn.

Teaching questions for EBM in real-time

Note that teaching question-asking skills can be integrated with any other clinical teaching, right at the bedside or other site of patient care,

---

Table 1.3 Key steps in teaching how to ask questions for EBM

1. **Recognize**: how to identify combinations of a patient's needs and a learner's needs that represent opportunities for the learner to build good questions.
2. **Select**: how to select from the recognized opportunities the one (or few) that best fits the needs of the patient and the learner at that clinical moment.
3. **Guide**: how to guide the learner in transforming knowledge gaps into well-built clinical questions.
4. **Assess**: how to assess the learner's performance and skill at asking pertinent, answerable clinical questions for practicing EBM.

and it needn't take much additional time. Modeling question-asking takes less than a minute, while coaching learners on asking a question about a patient usually takes 2–3 minutes.

Once we have formulated an important question with our learners, how might we keep track of it and follow its progress toward a clinically useful answer? In addition to the methods for saving questions we mentioned earlier, one tactic we've used for teaching questions is the "Educational Prescription", shown in Figure 1.2. These help both teachers and learners in five ways:

1. It specifies the clinical problem that generated the questions.

2. It states the question, in all of its key elements.

3. It specifies who is responsible for answering it.

4. It reminds everyone of the deadline for answering it (taking into account the urgency of the clinical problem that generated it).

5. Finally, it reminds everyone of the steps of searching, critically appraising, and relating the answer back to the patient.

How might we use the educational prescription in our clinical teaching? The number of ways is limited only by our imaginations and our opportunities for teaching. As we'll reinforce in Chapter 8, educational prescriptions have been incorporated into familiar in-patient teaching settings from work rounds and attending/consultant rounds to morning reports and noon conferences. They have also been used in outpatient teaching settings, such as the ambulatory morning report. You can download these forms from the accompanying CD and website.

Will you and your learners follow through on the educational prescriptions? You might, if you build the writing and "dispensing" of them into your everyday routine. One tactic we use is to make specifying clinical questions an integral part of presenting a new patient to the group. For example, we ask learners on our general medicine inpatient clinical teams, when presenting new patients, to tell us "31 things in 3 minutes" about each admission, although only the first 21 at the bedside. As shown in Table 1.4, the final element of their presentation is the specification of an important question to which they need to know the answer and don't. If the answer is vital to the immediate care of the patient, it can be provided at once by another member of the clinical team, perhaps by accessing some of the evidence synopsis resources you will learn more about in Chapter 2. Most of the time, the answer can wait a few hours or days, so the question can serve as the start of an educational prescription.

R̽ Educational Prescription

Patient's Name	Learner:

3-part Clinical Question

Target Disorder:

Intervention (+/– comparison):

Outcome:

Date and place to be filled:

Presentations will cover:
1. search strategy;
2. search results;
3. the validity of this evidence;
4. the importance of this valid evidence;
5. can this valid, important evidence be applied to your patient;
6. your evaluation of this process.

Figure 1.2 Educational Prescription form.

Table 1.4 A bedside patient presentation that includes an educational prescription

---

1. The patient's surname
2. The patient's age
3. When the patient was admitted
4. The illness or symptom(s) that led to admission. For each symptom, mention:
   5. Where in the body it is located
   6. Its quality
   7. Its quantity, intensity, and degree of impairment
   8. Its chronology: when it began, constant/episodic, progressive
   9. Its setting: under what circumstances did it/does it occur.
   10. Any aggravating or alleviating factors
   11. Any associated symptoms
12. Whether a similar problem had occurred previously. If so:
   13. How it was investigated
   14. What the patient was told about its cause
   15. How the patient had been treated for it
16. Pertinent past history of other conditions that are of diagnostic, prognostic or pragmatic significance and would affect the evaluation or treatment of the present illness
17. And how those other conditions have been treated
18. Family history, if pertinent to present illness or hospital care
19. Social history, if pertinent to present illness or hospital care
20. The condition on admission:
   a. Acutely and/or chronically ill
   b. Severity of complaints
   c. Requesting what sort of help
21. The pertinent physical findings on admission

And, after leaving the bedside and moving to a private location, finish with:

22. The pertinent diagnostic test results
23. Your concise, one-sentence problem synthesis statement
24. What you think is the most likely diagnosis ("leading hypothesis")
25. What few other diagnoses you're pursuing ("active alternatives")
26. The further diagnostic studies you plan to confirm the leading hypothesis or exclude active alternatives
27. Your estimate of the patient's prognosis
28. Your plans for treatment and counseling
29. How you will monitor the treatment in follow-up
30. Your contingency plans if the patient doesn't respond to initial treatment
31. The educational prescription you would like to write for yourself in order to better understand the patient's disorder (background knowledge) or how to care for the patient (foreground knowledge) in order to become a better clinician

---

Finally, we can ask our learners to write educational prescriptions for us. This role reversal can help in four ways:

1. The learners must supervise our question building, thereby honing their skills further.

2. The learners see us admitting our own knowledge gaps and practicing what we preach.

3. It adds fun to rounds and sustains group morale.

4. Our learners begin to prepare for their later roles as clinical teachers.

Like most clinical skills, learning to ask answerable questions for EBM takes time, coaching, and deliberate practice.[19] Our experience suggests that after a brief introduction, it takes supervising our learners' practice and giving them specific feedback on their questions to help them develop proficiency. Others have found that providing a brief introduction alone may not be sufficient for learners to show proficiency.[20]

That concludes this chapter on the first step in practicing and teaching EBM: asking answerable clinical questions. Since you and your learners will want to move quickly from asking questions to finding their answers, our next chapter will address this second step in practicing and teaching EBM.

References

1. Smith R. What clinical information do doctors need? *BMJ*. 1996;313(7064):1062–1068.

2. Dawes M, Sampson U. Knowledge management in clinical practice: a systematic review of information seeking behavior in physicians. *Int J Med Inf*. 2003;71(1):9–15.

3. Case DO. *Looking for information: A survey of research on information seeking, needs, and behavior*. San Diego: Academic Press; 2002.

4. Richardson WS. Ask, and ye shall retrieve (EBM note). *Evid Based Med*. 1998;3:100–101.

5. Oxman AD, Sackett DL, Guyatt GH, for the Evidence-Based Medicine Working Group. Users' guides to the medical literature. I. How to get started. *JAMA*. 1993;270(17):2093–2095.

6. Richardson WS, Wilson MC, Nishikawa J, et al. The well-built clinical question: a key to evidence-based decisions (editorial). *ACP J Club*. 1995;123(3):A12–A13.

7. Neighbour R. *The inner apprentice: an awareness-centred approach to vocational training for general practice*. Newbury: Petroc Press; 1996.

8. Schon DA. *Educating the reflective practitioner*. San Francisco: Jossey-Bass; 1987.

9. Claxton G. *Wise-up: the challenge of lifelong learning*. New York: Bloomsbury; 1999.

10. Richardson WS, Burdette SD. Practice corner: Taking evidence in hand (editorial). *ACP J Club*. 2003;138(1):A9.

11. Villanueva EV, Burrows EA, Fennessy PA, et al. Improving question formulation for use in evidence appraisal in a tertiary care setting: a randomised controlled trial. *BMC Med Inform Decis Mak*. 2001;1:4.

12. Cabell CH, Schardt C, Sanders L, et al. Resident utilization of information technology. *J Gen Intern Med*. 2001;16(12):838–844.

13. Booth A, O'Rourke AJ, Ford NJ. Structuring the pre-search interview: a useful technique for handling clinical questions. *Bull Med Libr Assoc*. 2000;88(3):239–246.

14. Rosenberg WM, Deeks J, Lusher A, et al. Improving searching skills and evidence retrieval. *J R Coll Phys London*. 1998;32(6):557–563.

15. Bergus GR, Randall CS, Sinift SD, et al. Does the structure of clinical questions affect the outcome of curbside consultations with specialty colleagues? *Arch Fam Med*. 2000;9(6):541–547.

16. Brassey J, Elwyn G, Price C, et al. Just in time information for clinicians: a questionnaire evaluation of the ATTRACT project. *BMJ*. 2001;322(7285):529–530.

17. Jerome RN, Giuse NB, Gish KW, et al. Information needs of clinical teams: analysis of questions received by the Clinical Informatics Consult Service. *Bull Med Libr Assoc*. 2001;89(2):177–184.

18. McGowan J, Hogg W, Campbell, et al. Just-in-time information improved decision-making in primary care: A randomized trial. *PLoS One*. 2008;3(11):e3785.

19. Ericsson KA. Deliberate practice and the acquisition and maintenance of expert performance in medicine and related domains. *Acad Med*. 2004;79(10):S70–S81.

20. Wyer PC, Naqvi Z, Dayan PS, et al. Do workshops in evidence-based practice equip participants to identify and answer questions requiring consideration of clinical research? A diagnostic skill assessment. *Adv Health Sci Educ*. 2009;14(4):515–533.

1

2 Acquiring the evidence: How to find current best evidence *and have current best evidence find us**

My students are dismayed when I say to them, "Half of what you are taught as medical students will in 10 years have been shown to be wrong. And the trouble is, none of your teachers knows which half."

Dr Sydney Burwell, Dean of Harvard Medical School[1]

As highlighted in the Introduction, keeping up-to-date with current best evidence for the care of our patients is challenging. As Dr Burwell's quote from over half a century ago (1956) indicates, new medical knowledge is evolving quite quickly. In the past two decades, the pace has accelerated because of the maturation of the spectrum of methods for biomedical research (from bench to bedside), and huge new investments in health-care research of over US$100 billion per year.

One solution for the problem of obsolescence of professional education is "problem-based learning" or "learning by inquiry". That is, when confronted by a clinical question for which we are unsure of the current best answer, developing the habit of looking for the current best answer as efficiently as possible. (Literary critics will point out the redundancy of the term "current best" – we risk their scorn to emphasize that last year's best answer may not be this year's.)

The success of learning by inquiry depends heavily on being able to find the current best evidence to manage pressing clinical problems, a task that can be either quick and highly rewarding or time-consuming and frustrating. Which of these it is depends on several factors that we can control or influence, including which questions we ask, how we ask these questions (see Ch. 1), how well we use information resources (the subject of this chapter), and how skilled we are in interpreting and applying these resources (detailed in the chapters that follow).

---

*Disclaimer: The lead author for this chapter is Brian Haynes, who developed or contributed to many of the resources described herein.

We can learn a great deal about current best information sources from librarians and other experts in medical informatics, and should seek hands-on training from them as an essential part of our clinical education. This chapter provides adjunctive strategies for clinicians to use to find evidence quickly – including some that we may not learn from librarians – as well as dealing with evidence that finds us, bidden or unbidden.

Here, we consider finding evidence to help solve clinical problems about the treatment or prevention, diagnosis and differential diagnosis, prognosis and clinical prediction, cause, and economics of a clinical problem. Fortuitously, both search ("pull") and alerting ("push") tools have greatly improved since the previous edition of this book and are becoming more comprehensive in their clinical scope.

"*Pre-appraised evidence*" resources are built according to an explicit process that values research according to its scientific merit ("hierarchy of research methods") and clinical relevance. The finest of these resources provide further processing by sorting evidence into *pre-appraised* and non-pre-appraised, and also sorting pre-appraised evidence according to a "6S" hierarchy (described below) that reflects its likelihood of direct usefulness to clinical practice decisions. The term "*pre-appraised*" evidence is emphasized here for three key reasons: if we don't know how to critically appraise research evidence, don't consistently apply the criteria, or don't have the time to do our own detailed critical appraisal, then we can look for answers in pre-appraised evidence resources. If we can't find what we want there, we need to tackle the harder task of searching larger bibliographic databases such as Medline and applying the critical appraisal skills that are taught in this book.

This chapter provides an orientation to the types of pre-appraised evidence sources that exist today, followed by "raw" evidence services (such as Medline). Then we provide opportunities to try your own hand at tracking down the best evidence-based answers to specific clinical problems.

Orientation to evidence-based information resources: where to find the best evidence

1. Burn your traditional textbooks

We begin with textbooks, only to dismiss all but the best of a new breed of them. If the pages of textbooks smelled like decomposing garbage when they became outdated, the non-smelly bits could be useful, because textbooks are often well organized for clinical use and much of their content could be current at any one time. Unfortunately, in most texts, there's no way to tell what information is up-to-date and what is not, or whether the information is evidence-based or simply expertise-based. (Expertise is essential in authoring recommendations for clinical care, but it is not enough to ensure that the recommendations are also "evidence-based" – this chapter provides ways to determine if the text you are reading is also evidence-based.) So, although we may find some useful information in texts about "background questions" (see Ch. 1), such as the pathophysiology of clinical problems, it is best not to use texts for seeking the answers to "foreground questions", such as the causal (risk) factors, diagnosis, prognosis, prevention or treatment of a disorder, unless they are also evidence-based and up-to-date.

Here's a 2-step screening test for whether a text is likely to be evidence-based and up-to-date:

1. A text that provides recommendations for patient care must have "in line" references to evidence that supports each of its key recommendations about the diagnosis, treatment, or prognosis of patients.

2. If the text does indicate exact references for its recommendations, check the date of publication of the references; if the most recent is more than 2–3 years old, you will need to check whether more recent studies require a change in recommendation.

Texts that fail these two screens should be used for background reading only, no matter how eminent their authors.

Table 2.1 provides a more detailed set of guides for the ideal text resource for clinical practice. Please note that the guides should only be applied to texts that are available online. Printed texts that include recommendations for tests and treatments cannot be reliably up-to-date because print production processes are too lengthy. Typically, it takes a year or more for print preparation before books begin shipping, and then the book continues to rot until the renewal process begins again, usually 2–4 years later. That's not to say that online texts are current either, let alone reliably evidence-based. Check out your favorites with the guides in Table 2.1. A text that scores less than 5 is definitely not "evidence-based" and should be used for "background" information at most.

Do you have any burning questions at this point? Here are three that you might have.

Table 2.1 Guides for assessing medical texts for evidence-based features

Criterion	Rating	
1. "In line references" for treatment recommendations *In line = references that are in the text next to individual declarations*	0 None or few	1 Usually or always
2. "In line references" for diagnostic recommendations	0 None or few	1 Usually or always
3. Policy indicating steps by the editors/authors to find new evidence *Likely to be found in the "About" information concerning the text*	0 Absent	1 Present
4. Policy indicating the quality rating of research evidence ("levels of evidence") 	0 Absent	1 Present
5. Policy indicating the grading of strength of recommendations ("grades of recommendations") 	0 Absent	1 Present
6. Date stamping of individual chapters *Should be at the beginning or end of each chapter*	0 Absent	1 Present
7. Indication of a schedule for updating chapters *Should be at the start of each chapter or in "About"*	0 Absent	1 Present
8. "New evidence" tabs for individual chapters/topics *Could be called "updates", "best new evidence", etc.*	0 Absent	1 Present
9. User alerts for new evidence according to user discipline *Can users sign up for alerts for updates for specific disciplines (e.g., primary care; cardiology)?*	0 Absent	1 Present
10. User alerts for new evidence according to individual topic *Can users sign up for new evidence alerts for specific topics (e.g., diabetes; warts; hypertension)?*	0 Absent	1 Present
11. Federated search of content and external evidence source *Simultaneous search of several identified evidence-based sources*	0 Absent	1 Present

©*Health Information Research Unit, McMaster University. Contact: Brian Haynes, e-mail: bhaynes@mcmaster.ca.*
Note: This survey is only for texts that are available online.

First, "What about authority?". If we added that as a criterion for rating a text, it could go along these lines: "Does the publication include a list of distinguished editors who are elderly white males with endowed chairs at prestigious institutions?" Just joking – we believe, high fidelity, explicit processes for finding, evaluating, incorporating, and updating evidence concerning the diagnosis, course, cause, prevention, treatment, and rehabilitation of health problems are more important than named chairs. It's not that expertise isn't important, but even if named chairs do connote expertise at some time in a person's career, the chair-holder is more likely to be renowned for the research they do than the care they provide, or will be so sub-specialized and out of touch with level of care provided by frontline clinicians, that his advice is of dubious value for handling all but the most complicated and arcane cases, which we would need to refer in any event. We like to look at what's under the hood, not at the ornaments atop it. Authority comes from an explicit, robust evidence process.

Second, "Do we really mean that traditional textbooks should be burned?". We do (and not even recycled – they should be incinerated as dangerous waste). At this point, our publisher is probably getting edgy about where this discussion is heading, considering all the journals and textbooks they publish, including this one. Any money saved from not purchasing traditional textbooks can be spent on better sources of current best knowledge for clinical practice.

Third, "What's the alternative to traditional, expertise-based textbooks of medicine?". Answer: "Evidence-based, regularly updated, online texts and pre-appraised evidence services." Read on, as we head into the "6S" territory of evidence-based resources.

2. Take a "6S" approach to evidence-based information access*

Practical resources to support evidence-based healthcare decisions are rapidly evolving. New and better services are being created through the combined forces of increasing numbers of clinically important studies, more robust evidence synthesis and synopsis services, and better information technology. You can help yourself to current best evidence by recognizing and using the most evolved information services for the topics of interest to you and your patients.

---

*With permission from the American College of Physicians, this section draws heavily on DiCenso et al. 2009.[2]

Examples

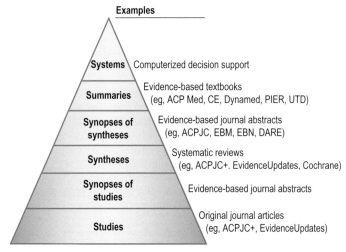

Figure 2.1 The "6S" hierarchy of organization of pre-appraised evidence. (Reprinted from DiCenso et al. 2009, with permission from the American College of Physicians.)[2] ACP Med, *ACP Medicine*; CE, *Clinical Evidence*; PIER, *Physicians Education and Information Resource*; UTD, *UpToDate*; ACPJC, *ACP Journal Club*; EBM, *Evidence-Based Medicine*; EBN, *Evidence-Based Nursing*; DARE, *Database of Reviews of Evidence*.

Figure 2.1 provides a 6-level hierarchical structure, with original "studies" at the base, "synopses" of the most clinically relevant studies just above the base, "syntheses" (systematic reviews) of evidence just above, topped by "synopses" of the premier syntheses, then clinical topic "summaries", and, at the pinnacle, the most evolved evidence-based information "systems" that link evidence-based recommendations with individual patients. *You should begin your search for best evidence by looking at the highest-level resource available for the problem that prompts your search.* The details of how to do this follow.

Systems

The ideal. A perfect evidence-based clinical information *system* would integrate and concisely summarize all relevant and important research evidence about a clinical problem and would automatically link, through an electronic medical record, a specific patient's circumstances to the relevant information. We would then consult – indeed, be prompted by – the system whenever the patient's medical record is reviewed. The information contained in the system would be based on an explicit review process for finding and evaluating new evidence as it is published and then reliably and promptly updated whenever important new, high-quality, confirmatory or discordant research evidence becomes available. The clinician and patient could therefore always have the benefit of the current best evidence.

It is important to note that such a system would not tell decision-makers what to do. These judgments need to integrate the system's evidence with the patient's circumstances and wishes via the practitioner's experience and clinical expertise.[3] The system's role would be to ensure that the cumulative research evidence concerning the patient's problem is immediately at hand. Further, to maximize speed of use, our first point of interaction would be a short *synopsis*, but links to *syntheses* and then to original *studies* would be provided so that we could drill down as deeply as needed to verify the accuracy, currency, applicability and details of the synopsis.

The present state of evolution. Current systems don't reach this level of perfection as yet, but production models exist for parts of such systems. Electronic medical record systems with computerized decision support rules have been shown in randomized trials to improve the process and sometimes the outcome of care.[4] However, these systems cover a limited range of clinical problems, are not necessarily based on current best evidence, and are mainly "homebuilt" and not easily transferred to most practice settings. Further, more recent studies have suggested unanticipated adverse events associated with their implementation highlighting the complexity of this issue. Thus, the jury is still out as to whether computerized decision support will be a panacea or even a net benefit for evidence-based care.

Summaries (exemplar *Summary* publications are described in alphabetical order by title)

Some excellent, but less-developed, summaries of evidence for individual clinical problems are readily available. There are several leading contenders with overlapping clinical content. *Clinical Evidence* from the BMJ Group (www.clinicalevidence.com[†]) is a pace-setter for

[†]In the wild world of the internet, URLs often change. If this or any other URL in the book doesn't work, "Google" the title of the publication (go to www.google.com and put the title in the search line) and you will likely find the new URL; also, if you work for an institution that has an electronic library, be sure to check to see if any of the *Summary* texts are in its licensed collection.

scientific rigor and updating and has an expanding repertoire of topics for general medicine, including many common clinical problems. Its reviews of evidence adhere to high scientific standards and it posts newly published evidence in an update table for each topic, so that readers are not left wondering if the review is up-to-date. Its topic list is finite, but is expanded by a "federated" search process that retrieves not only its own content but pre-appraised references for other topics as well. It is limited to coverage of therapy topics unlike the other resources mentioned in this section, which have a broader coverage. The *Physicians Information and Education Resource*, PIER (http://pier. acponline.org/index.html), has an evidence-based approach with topics mainly of interest to primary care practice. *Dynamed* (www.ebsco-host.com/dynamed) has a robust evidence-based infrastructure, and a broad topic coverage, but a less formal approach to summarizing evidence. *UpToDate* on DVD and the web (www.uptodate.com), is updated semi-annually (with some unscheduled interim updates), extensively referenced, often with key study descriptions, and also provides MEDLINE abstracts for key evidence. This provides the user with at least a sporting chance of dating and appraising the supporting evidence. *UpToDate* lacks a formal appraisal process for evidence coming into the text but is slowly implementing a grading process for evidence that its authors choose to present.

Several additional textbooks of medicine are in the process of upgrading their evidence infrastructure, reflecting a more rigorous process for seeking and using evidence, including *ACP Medicine* (www.acpmedicine. com), *ACS Surgery* (www.acssurgery.com), *eTherapeutics* (www. e-therapeutics.ca), *Harrison's Practice* (www.harrisonspractice.com/ practice/ub), and *First Consult* (www.mdconsult.com/php/142221516–2/ homepage).

We look forward to many more such texts soon; but beware, these texts are in transition. It is important to check whether the systematic consideration of evidence promised in the title and introduction of these books is actually delivered in the content. Unfortunately, the term "evidence-based" has been adopted by many publishers and authors without the savvy or scruples to deliver honest evidence-based content. Thus, your first task in seeking evidence-based summaries is to look for texts and websites that pass the screening tests above and the majority of the guides in Table 2.1.

Although none of the *Summary* publications described above is integrated with individual-patient electronic medical records (EMRs), they can be run through the same computers that run EMRs and even within

EMRs, so that one need not go to a remote location to find them. Even when best evidence from research is immediately juxtaposed to the clinical record, however, connecting the right information to a specific patient's problems requires that we understand evidence-based care principles and that we apply skill and judgment in using the resources. Fortunately, these evolving *Summary* resources can reduce the burdens considerably if they have adequate, ongoing evidence-processing.

Some internet-based "aggregators" provide a special "6S supermarket" service for evidence-based information. Ovid, for example, provides access to a huge collection of texts, journals, and databases, including summaries such as *Clinical Evidence*, while STAT!Ref includes *PIER, ACP Medicine*, and searches of most of the "S" levels below. Ovid's *Evidence-Based Medicine Reviews* (EBMR) provides access to the Cochrane Library, *ACP Journal Club*, the *Database of Abstracts of Reviews of Evidence* (DARE), and MEDLINE, all in an integrated format that permits tracking from, for example, a full-text original article to a synopsis that describes it, a synthesis (systematic review) in which it is incorporated, and related articles on the same topic. Later in this chapter, we'll review some other "federated" search services that retrieve information from many sources simultaneously, including leading evidence-based ones.

The *Summary* publications mentioned here are but a few of those available today. If your discipline or clinical question isn't mentioned, consult the more complete listing in the accompanying EBM 4/e CD, or try SCHARR (www.shef.ac.uk/scharr/ir/netting) or Google (www.google.com; put "evidence-based" on Google's search line followed by your discipline or the clinical problem you are researching, e.g., evidence-based warts).

Synopses of syntheses

Synopses are carefully edited, typically one-page, structured descriptions of pre-appraised articles that report sound research with clinically relevant and newsworthy findings. They appear in such publications as *ACP Journal Club* (www.acpjc.org), *Evidence-Based Mental Health* (http://ebmh.bmj.com), and DARE, the *Database of Abstracts of Reviews of Evidence* (www.crd.york.ac.uk/crdweb). Synopses come in two flavors, *synopses of syntheses* (i.e., of systematic reviews) and synopses of articles reporting original studies. *Synopses of syntheses* are higher in the hierarchy (Figure 2.1) because syntheses review all pertinent studies concerning an intervention, diagnostic test, prognosis or etiology, whereas original articles describe just one study.

When no current, adequate evidence-based *summary* exists for a clinical problem, then *synopses of syntheses* are the next best source. What busy practitioner has time to assemble and review the available evidence on her own or wade through a 70-page Cochrane review? Although these detailed articles and reviews are essential building blocks for current best knowledge, they are often too heavy to lift on the run. Synopses do a lot of the heavy lifting for us.

The perfect synopsis would provide only, and exactly, enough information to support a clinical action. The declarative title for each abstract that appears in *ACP Journal Club*, and *Evidence-Based Mental Health* (we'll describe these evidence-based journals later in this chapter) represents an attempt at this. Here's an example: "Review: Brand-name drugs are not more effective than generic versions for treating cardiovascular disease".[5] In some circumstances, this title provides enough information to allow the decision-maker either to proceed, assuming familiarity with the nature of the intervention and its alternatives, or to look further for the details, which, for ideal synopses, are immediately at hand. The full abstract for this item is in *ACP Journal Club*, with an abstract and commentary on one printed page, accessible in the original print issue or electronically. Electronic access is definitely the best way to go for all these resources (more about that later).

Syntheses

If more detail is needed or no synopsis is at hand, then databases of systematic reviews (syntheses) are available. Syntheses are based on exhaustive searches for evidence, explicit scientific reviews of the studies uncovered in the search, and systematic assembly of the evidence, to provide as clear a signal about the effects of a healthcare intervention as the accumulated evidence will allow. The Cochrane Collaboration provides the largest single source of synopses, about 30–40% of the world's supply. Cochrane Reviews have mainly focused on preventive or therapeutic interventions to date, but the Cochrane Collaboration started summarizing diagnostic test evidence.

A key single source of pre-appraised syntheses is *EvidenceUpdates* (http://plus.mcmaster.ca/EvidenceUpdates), a free service sponsored by the BMJ Group. *EvidenceUpdates* includes all Cochrane Reviews, systematic reviews from over 120 clinical journals, and syntheses commissioned by the US Agency for Healthcare Research and Quality, the Canadian Agency for Drugs and Technologies in Health, and the UK National Health Service Health Technology Assessments. Other ready sources of syntheses are the *Database of Reviews of Evidence*, DARE (free at www.crd.york.ac.uk/crdweb) and The Cochrane Library, which includes Cochrane Reviews and *DARE* and is available on a quarterly CD, the internet (www 3.interscience.wiley.com/cgi-bin/mrwhome/106568753/ HOME), and Ovid's EBMR service.

Additional reviews not available in the preceding sources, and typically of lower quality, can be found in bibliographic databases such as PubMed and EMBASE. For both of these, searches are likely to be more productive, with less "junk", using the "Clinical Queries" search strategy for "reviews". Obtained by this route, the searcher must take on the responsibility for critical appraisal of the retrieved articles (see Ch. 3).

Synopses of studies

If none of the higher levels yields the answer to a problem you are interested in, then *synopses of studies* is the next level to check. These are the same as synopses of syntheses described above, except that reports of individual studies are described. Synopses of studies appear in the same publications (*ACPJC, EBN*) and provide structured abstracts of individual, high quality studies, that is, studies that not only meet basic critical appraisal criteria, but also are selected for clinical relevance and interest.

Studies

It takes time to summarize new evidence, and summaries, synopses and syntheses necessarily follow the publication of original *studies*, usually by at least 6 months, and sometimes by years. If every other "S" fails (i.e. no systems, summaries, synopses, or syntheses exist with clear answers to your question), then it's time to look for original studies. Looking for these in full-text print journals (the classic way of "keeping up-to-date"), is generally hopeless but pre-appraised studies can be retrieved relatively efficiently on the internet in several ways.

Fortunately, several new "evidence refinery" services have become available since the third edition of this book. Most of these article critical appraisal services are organized according to a targeted range of clinical disciplines, such as general practice (*Essential Evidence Plus*, www.essentialevidenceplus.com; requires a subscription); primary care, internal medicine and subspecialties (*ACPJC+*; http://plus.mcmaster. ca/acpjc; membership benefit of the American College of Physicians); general medicine and major specialties (*EvidenceUpdates*, http://plus. mcmaster.ca/EvidenceUpdates; sponsored by BMJ Group); nursing (*Best*

Evidence for Nursing Care, http://plus.mcmaster.ca/np; sponsored by the Health Information Research Unit, McMaster University); and rehabilitation sciences (*Rehab PLUS*; http://plus.mcmaster.ca/rehab; sponsored by the Health Information Research Unit, McMaster University). These services also provide "alerts" for newly published evidence according to your clinical discipline, an important complement to being able to search for evidence, helping to fill the gaps of "what you don't know but didn't think to ask" and "what you know that ain't so". Our recommendation is to subscribe to or register for, and get to know, the service that best matches your information needs.

General search engines

> **Warning**: you are now entering "do it yourself" appraisal territory!

If you don't know which database is best suited to your question, "meta" search engines tuned for healthcare content can assemble access across a number of web-based services. At least two of these search engines include some attention to issues of quality of evidence by segmenting the search yield according to source (including several of the pre-appraisal services mentioned above). These "federated" search engines are SUMSearch (http://sumsearch.uthscsa.edu) and TRIP, Turning Research into Practice (www.tripdatabase.com/index.html), both of which are free to users. Nevertheless, users must verify that the source of a given retrieved item is evidence-based, or appraise the individual items identified by such a search to determine which are based on sound evidence.

If the search is for a treatment, then the Cochrane Library includes the Cochrane Central Register of Controlled Trials (CENTRAL), also available as part of *EBMR* on Ovid, where it is integrated with *ACP Journal Club* and *DARE*. But all these services are subject to the timeline required for evidence summarization, to which is added the Ovid timeline for electronic posting and integration, and appraisal of the individual items by the searcher is essential if the source is not one of the pre-appraisal services.

For original articles and reviews hot off the press, MEDLINE is freely available (www.ncbi.nlm.nih.gov/PubMed), and the Clinical Queries screen (available as a menu item on the main PubMed screen or directly at www.ncbi.nlm.nih.gov/entrez/query/static/clinical.html) provides detailed search strategies that home in on clinical content for therapy, diagnosis, prognosis, clinical prediction, etiology, economics, and systematic reviews. These search strategies are embedded in the Clinical Queries screen, so that you don't need to remember them. You can use the "sensitive" search strategy if you want to retrieve every article that might bear on your question. Or you can use the "specific" search strategy if you want "a few good references" and don't have time to sort out the citations that aren't on target. In either case, although the CQ filters improve the yield of high quality clinical-relevant evidence, you must do your own critical appraisal of individual articles.

These search strategies can also be run in proprietary systems that include the MEDLINE database, although they need some translation for the search syntax that is unique to each system. A complete listing of the search strategies for various access routes and databases appears on: http://hiru.mcmaster.ca/hiru/HIRU_Hedges_home.aspx.

If you still have no luck and the topic is, say, a new treatment (that one of your patients has asked about but you don't yet know about …), then you can try Google (www.google.com). You can retrieve a product monograph in a few milliseconds in which you'll find what the manufacturer of the treatment claims it can do along with detailed information on adverse effects, contraindications, and prescribing. You can also retrieve open access summaries, for example, from eMedicine, but these are not as yet reliably evidence-based or up-to-date. Many original studies and syntheses are also available via Google, but the quick retrieval times for millions of documents is counterbalanced by the burden of appraisal that is required to determine which of these documents accurately represents current best evidence. That said, Google is the fastest way to get to almost any service on the internet that you haven't "bookmarked" for your web browser, including all the ones named in this article that are web-accessible: just type in their proper names and you'll likely "get lucky". We'd like to note here that one of our colleagues, Ann McKibbon found in a small study that it was not uncommon for physicians to change from a correct decision to a wrong decision about a clinical scenario following completion of a search – but this was associated with the search engine used – in particular, Google was a likely contributor to wrong answers.

3. Organize access to evidence-based information services

It's worth emphasizing that almost all the resources just reviewed are available on the internet. The added value of accessing these services on the internet is considerable, including links to full-text journal articles, patient information, and complementary texts. To be able to do this, you need to be in a location, such as a medical library, hospital or clinic, where all the necessary licenses have been obtained, or, better still, have proxy server permission or remote access to a local computer from whatever organizations to which you belong, whether it be a university, hospital or professional corporation, so that you can use these services wherever you plug your computer into the internet. A typical package of services for health professionals might include an Ovid collection of full-text journals, *EBMR*, *Clinical Evidence*, *Dynamed*, *UpToDate* and STAT!Ref for *PIER*, *ACP Medicine*, and *ACS Surgery*.

You should ask your university, professional school, hospital, or clinic librarian about what digital library licenses are available and how you can tap into them. If you lack local institutional access, you may still be in luck, depending on the region in which you live. For example, some countries have national health libraries and some countries have licensed access to the Cochrane Library. Also, many professional societies provide access to some of the resources as membership benefits or at reduced rates.

Don't assume that your institution or professional society will make evidence-based choices about the publications and services it provides. You should decide which services you need for your clinical work and then check to see if these have been chosen by your institution. If not, make a case for the resources you want. When you do so, be prepared to indicate what your library could give up. The easiest targets for discontinuation are high-priced, low-impact-factor journals, and it will be perceived as a whole lot less self-serving if you target publications in your own clinical discipline that are at the bottom end of the evidence-based ladder of evolution, rather than the high-priced favorite journals of your colleagues in other disciplines. A guide for which journals to select for several disciplines appears in an article by Ann McKibbon and colleagues.[6]

If you live in a country with low resources, don't despair! The Health Internetwork Access to Research Information program (HINARI, www.healthInternetwork.net/) provides institutional access to a wide range of journals and texts at no or low cost.

If you are on your own, have no computer, can't afford to subscribe to journals, but have access to a public library with a computer linked to the internet, you're still in luck. Free access to high-quality evidence-based information abounds on the internet, beginning with EvidenceUpdates for pre-appraised evidence, TRIP and SUMsearch; open-access journals, such as the *BMJ* and *CMAJ*, BioMed Central (www.biomedcentral.com/), and the Public Library of Science (www.PLOS.org/); and the many evidence-based resources available through SCHARR (www.shef. ac.uk/~scharr/ir/netting/). Beware, however, that using free internet services requires a commitment to finding and appraising information unless using the pre-appraised services; free, high-quality evidence-based information is in much lower supply and concentration on the internet than in the specialized, evidence pre-appraisal resources mentioned above. The reason is simple: it is much easier and cheaper to produce low-quality, rather than high-quality, information.

4. Is it time to change how you seek best evidence?

Compare the 6S approach with how you usually seek evidence-based information. Is it time to revise your tactics? If, for example, it surprises you that MEDLINE (PUBMED) is low on the 6S list of resources for finding current best evidence, then this communication will have served a purpose. Resources for finding evidence are rapidly evolving, and searches can be a lot quicker and more satisfying for answering clinical questions if the features of your quest match those of one of the evolved services. This is no knock against MEDLINE, which continues to serve as a premier access route to the studies and reviews that form the foundation for all the other more specialized databases reviewed above. But big rewards can be gained from becoming familiar with pre-appraised evidence resources and using them whenever the right clinical question presents itself.

Another way to think of organizing your information needs, outlined by Muir Gray, is "prompt, pull, push". "Prompt" corresponds to the highest "S" level "systems". When you interact with an electronic patient record, or an evidence-based diagnostic or pharmacy service, it ought to prompt you if a feature of your patient corresponds to an evidence-based care guideline that you haven't already incorporated into their care plan. As indicated above, such systems are not widely available at present, although this is beginning to change. "Pull" corresponds to the lower 5 levels of the 6S approach: you go searching to "pull" the evidence you need from available resources. "Push" refers to having evidence sent to you; controlling this is the subject of the next section.

> To embrace the principles of evidence-based medicine, you need an operational plan for the regular use of both "push" and "pull" resources that are tailored as closely as possible to your discipline needs. Details about how to proceed follow.

How to deal with the evidence that finds you ("push" evidence): keeping up-to-date efficiently

1. Cancel your full-text journal subscriptions

Trying to keep current with the knowledge base that is pertinent to your clinical practice by reading full-text journals is a hopeless task. From an evidence-based perspective, for a broad discipline such as general practice or any major specialty (pediatrics, psychiatry, surgery), the number of articles you need to read to find one article that meets basic criteria for quality and relevance ranges from 86 to 107 for the top five full-text general journals.[6] At, say, 2 minutes per article, that's about 3 hours to find one article ready for clinical action; and then the article may cover old ground or provide "me-too" evidence of yet-another statin, or not be useful to you because of the way you have specialized your practice. You should trade in your (traditional) journal subscriptions. That will save you time but won't necessarily save you money, because you will need to invest in better resources for keeping current (see below).

2. Invest in evidence-based journals and online evidence services

During the past few years, the Health Information Research Unit at McMaster University has collaborated with professional organizations and publishers to create several online services that "push" new evidence to subscribers. Most of these services also archive evidence that can be "pulled" to provide best evidence concerning specific clinical questions. These services include *ACPJC+*, *EvidenceUpdates*, *Medscape Best Evidence Alerts* (WebMD), *Nursing PLUS*, and *Rehab PLUS*. For each of these, you can sign up according to your clinical interests and then will receive regular alerts to new studies that have been pre-appraised for scientific merit and clinical relevance. Relevance assessments are made by a voluntary international panel of physicians, nurses, and rehab practitioners. (If you are in independent clinical practice in medicine, nursing, or rehabilitation, you may wish to sign up as a rater: send an e-mail to: more@mcmaster.ca). Similar services exist for other disciplines, and by other providers, and you can use the Table 2.1 guides 3, 4, 9 and 10 to judge their credentials.

A number of periodicals summarize the better studies in traditional journals, making their selections according to explicit criteria for scientific merit, providing structured abstracts and expert commentaries about the context of the studies and the clinical applicability of their findings. These synoptic journals include *ACP Journal Club*, *Evidence-Based Medicine*, *Evidence-Based Mental Health*, *Evidence-Based Nursing*, *Evidence Based Child Health* and a few others. Synoptic journals do what traditional journals wish they could do, in selecting the best studies, finding the best articles from all relevant journals and summarizing them in one place. Traditional journals can't do this because they can only publish from among the articles that authors choose to send them.

If you find articles on a topic of high interest to you in an online evidence-based publication, and these appear in a journal to which you or your institution subscribes, then you can often invoke a number of ancillary services. For example, say you are interested in the *EBM* (http://ebm.bmj.com/) article, "Review: inhaled corticosteroids do not reduce mortality but increase pneumonia in COPD".[7] This synopsis is linked to the full-text article in *JAMA*, so you can read the full review. You can also "click" (1) to be alerted when new articles cite this review; (2) to be connected to similar synopses in EBM or to similar articles in the publisher's other journals; (3) to e-mail the item to a friend or colleague; or (4) to download the synopsis to citation manager software. The synopsis is also linked to the PubMed abstract of the original article and this leads to PubMed's various features, such as "Related Articles" and "Links" to other services.

For the most part, these evidence-based synopsis journals are targeted for generalists. However, subspecialty evidence-based journal clubs and books are sprouting on the web, such as PedsCCM *Evidence Based Journal Club* (http://pedsccm.org/EBJournal_Club_intro.php) for pediatrics and Evidence-Based Dermatology (www.blackwellpublishing.com/medicine/bmj/dermatology/), which is one of a collection of evidence-based specialty books. Googling "evidence-based [your discipline or topic of choice]" is a good way to find these resources. A better way is to search SCHARR, which provides links to a multitude of evidence-based services (www.shef.ac.uk/scharr/ir/netting/).

Walking the walk: searching for evidence to solve patient problems

As in swimming, bicycle riding, alligator wrestling, and flame eating, the use of evidence-based information resources is best learned by examples and practice, not by didactic instruction alone. Commit yourself to paper on the matters on the problem below before you move on to the rest of the chapter:

1. The key question to seek an answer for (using the PICO(T) guidelines from Ch. 1).

2. The best answer to the clinical problem that you currently have stored in your brain (being as quantitative as possible).

3. The evidence resources (both traditional and avant garde) that you would consult to find best current answers.

Clinical scenario

Mrs Smothers, an accountant, is an overweight, 56-year-old white woman with type 2 diabetes, first diagnosed 3 years ago. She visits you in a somewhat agitated state. She missed her previous appointment ("tax time"), and has not been at the clinic for over a year. Her 54-year-old sister also had diabetes and recently died of a heart attack. Mrs Smothers found some information on the internet that will allow her to calculate her own risk of heart attack but she lacks some of the information needed to do the calculation, including her cholesterol and recent hemoglobin A_{1c}. She wants your help in completing the calculation and your advice about reducing her risk.

She is currently trying to quit her smoking habit of 25 years. She is on a prescribed regimen of a calorie-restricted diet (with no weight loss in the past year), exercise (she states about 20 minutes of walking once or twice a week, hampered by her osteoarthritis), and metformin 1000 mg twice a day (sometimes missed, especially when she skips meals). Mr Smothers accompanies Mrs Smothers on this visit and interjects that she is also taking vitamin E and beta-carotene to lower her risk for heart disease, based on a "health advisory" that Mr Smothers read on the internet. The occasional fasting blood sugars she has taken recently have been between 7 and 14 mmol/L (126–252 mg/dL). She hasn't had an eye examination in over a year and didn't get a 'flu' shot last Fall. She has no other physical complaints at present, but admits to being depressed since her sister's death. She specifically denies symptoms of chest pain, stroke, or claudication.

On examination, Mrs Smothers is 98 kg (216 lb) in weight and 172 cm (5' 8") in height. Her blood pressure is 148/86 mmHg in the left arm with a large adult cuff, repeated. The rest of her examination is unremarkable, including her optic fundi, neuro, chest, cardiovascular system, abdomen, skin, and feet.

You ask her what risk calculator she found and she shows you the web page that she had printed out (http://betterdiabetescare.nih.gov/TOOLBOXrisk.htm). You tell her that you will check out the web page and enthusiastically endorse tightening up her regimen to bring her into the "green zone" for blood sugar, blood pressure and cholesterol control. She is not keen to consume additional prescription medications, preferring "natural remedies", but states that she is open to discussion, especially in view of her sister's death. She wants to know her risk of having a heart attack or stroke and just how much benefit she can expect from any additional medication you might propose for her. You tell her that you will be pleased to help her get the answers to her questions, but will need to update her lab tests and have her return in 2 weeks. She is not very pleased about having to wait, but accepts your explanation.

Heeding a recent dictum from your clinic manager, you order a "lean and mean" minimalist set of lab tests: a hemoglobin A_{1c}, lipid profile, creatinine, urinary micro albumin: creatinine ratio, and electrocardiogram. These investigations show that Mrs Smothers has an A_{1c} of 8.9% (normal range 4–6%), urinary albumin:creatinine ratio of 7.9 mg/mmol (normal <1.9), and hyperlipidemia, with total cholesterol 6.48 mmol/L (250 mg/dL; target <5.2 for primary prevention), LDL 3.4 mmol/L (131 mg/dL), HDL 0.9 mmol/L (34.7 mg/dL), and triglycerides 3.9 mmol/L (345 mg/dL; <1.7 (150) desirable).

2

Write down the key questions that identify the evidence needed to give Mrs Smothers clear answers about the cardiovascular risks from her condition and benefits from its treatments. Then indicate your best answers before searching (stick your neck out!), and select evidence resources that you feel will provide current best evidence to support your answers suited to this patient.

Questions:

Your initial answers:

Your proposed evidence resources:

At this point, you should have written down the key question(s), your top-of-the-head answer(s), and the evidence resources that you feel are best suited to answer these questions. Now would be a good time to try your hand at finding the answers by the routes you've selected, keeping track of how much time, ease/aggravation and money your searches cost and how satisfied you are in the end. Put yourself under some time pressure: summarize the best evidence you can find in 30 minutes or less for each question. (You may be thinking about skipping this exercise, hoping that the rest of this chapter will teach you how to do it effortlessly. But there is wisdom in the maxim "no pain, no gain".) Invest at least 30 minutes of your time on at least one of the questions before you press on. (As a teaching tip here, sometimes we give each member of our team a different evidence resource to search for the answer to the same clinical question. We find this to be a fun way of comparing and contrasting search strategies and evidence resources.)

What follows is based on the general approach, described at the beginning of this chapter, to identifying and using key evidence-based resources. It is important to note that there may be more than one good route (not to mention a myriad of bad routes), and that, as this book ages, better routes will assuredly be built. Indeed, many improved resources have become available since publication of the third edition of this book in 2005, and resources such as *EBMR*, *Clinical Evidence*, and the Cochrane Library, have greatly matured. Thus, one of the foundations of providing efficient, evidence-based healthcare is keeping tabs on the availability, scope and quality of new resources that are directly pertinent to our own professional practice.

If you have tried to search for evidence on these problems, compare what you did and what you found with our methods. If you haven't tried to search yet, we issue you a challenge: see if you can find a better answer than we did (we searched in mid-2009, but we will applaud you for a better answer that you found after this time; we hope and expect that the evidence will keep improving).

Carrying out the searching steps

Basic steps for acquiring the evidence to support a clinical decision are shown in Figure 2.2. We've supplied the clinical problem, and have asked you to take the first step, defining the questions to be answered, following the lead in Chapter 1. Have a go at it if you haven't done so already. Here's our try for the example above.

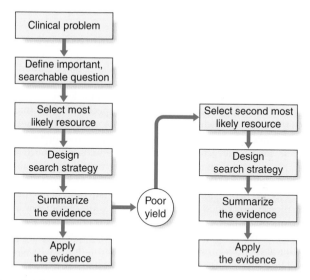

Figure 2.2 General search strategy.

Problem

Type 2 diabetes and related cardiovascular risk.

Step 1. Asking answerable questions

Based on the information at hand, we posed several questions. First, from the patient's primary motivation for visiting, "In a 56-year-old woman with poorly controlled type 2 diabetes mellitus, microproteinuria, elevated blood pressure, and dyslipidemia, what is the evidence concerning increased risk for cardiovascular complications?" Second, among such patients, does "tight" or intensive control of glucose, blood pressure, cholesterol, and proteinuria reduce subsequent morbidity and mortality, compared with lesser levels of control? Third, compared with placebo or no intervention, what is the evidence that beta-carotene and vitamin E supplements reduce cardiovascular risk among people who are at elevated cardiovascular risk but have not experienced cardiovascular events (i.e., primary prevention)?

Step 2A. Selecting an evidence resource

Step 2A is to decide where and how to search. Such a patient would often be seen in primary care, internal medicine, and endocrinology, so the focus should be on the best and quickest evidence-based information sources for these clinical disciplines, including general and specialized bibliographic databases, in both print and electronic form.

Electronic media with periodic updates (especially on the internet, with CD/DVD valuable when the internet is not readily accessible) have rendered paper sources obsolete for looking up current best evidence. Electronic media are generally much more accessible, much more thoroughly searchable, and, most importantly, have the potential to be much more up-to-date than paper-based resources. Moreover, hypertext and the internet permit unlimited linkages to related and supplementary information. Thus, a good computer (whether yours or someone else's) with an internet link (or at least a CD-ROM/DVD drive), and a working knowledge of the evidence resources that have been developed for our own clinical discipline, can make an important difference to whether you will be successful in becoming an evidence-based practitioner.

How to deal with the evidence that finds you

The first piece of information to consider in this case falls into the general category of "evidence that finds you"; as in our case, patients sometimes find information that they want you to comment on, so you need an efficient approach to evaluating the pedigree and evidence base for claims they encounter on the internet or other media. This patient brought along a web page (http://betterdiabetescare.nih.gov/TOOLBOXrisk.htm) that she had found through Google, so it was easy to examine this source. This website has impeccable credentials, with material prepared by the National Diabetes Education Program with sponsorship from the US National Institutes of Health, the National Institute of Diabetes and Digestive and Kidney Diseases, and Centers for Disease Control, and has no commercial advertising. This is not to say that the information on the website is necessarily either accurate or up-to-date, but it is more likely to be so than websites that lack these features. You breathe a sigh of relief for such an easy search.

Three risk calculators for cardiovascular disease are offered on the website, one from Framingham in the US (http://hp2010.nhlbihin.net/atpiii/calculator.asp?usertype=prof), and two from the UK, the most specific of which calculates risk of developing cardiovascular disease among people with type 2 diabetes (www.dtu.ox.ac.uk/index.php?maindoc=/riskengine/). All are supported by published studies. Because the UK calculator was specifically developed among patients with diabetes and is more recent, you retrieve the relevant study cited.[8] Details in this report indicate that the patients were an "inception cohort" of 4540 newly diagnosed patients with type 2 diabetes mellitus, followed for a median of over 10 years, with close monitoring for cardiovascular and other complications, and with very few patients being lost to follow-up or having missing data. As you will learn in Chapter 4, these features mean that the study meets critical appraisal criteria for the validity of prognostic studies. You decide to download the risk calculator to your computer and fire it up. You plug in the lab results for Mrs Smothers and the display is as shown in Figure 2.3.

According to the UKPDS risk calculator, Mrs Smothers has a substantial absolute risk (24.2%) of experiencing coronary heart disease (CHD) during the coming decade. The calculator allows you to modify the figures, monitoring your patient's status over time as test results change, and estimating the effect of interventions that alter the lab results and blood pressure. Keeping our skeptic's hat on, however, we quickly checked

2

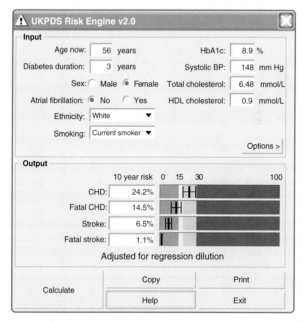

Figure 2.3 UKPDS cardiovascular risk calculator for patients with Type 2 diabetes mellitus.

EvidenceUpdates and found a study comparing UKPDS and Framingham cardiovascular risk estimates in an independent population with type 2 diabetes in Australia.[9] UKPDS performed "reasonably well" (Framingham did not) in identifying those at high cardiovascular risk, but considerably overestimated the observed event CHD rates. The authors speculate that this could be due to different populations or better treatments these days. We can provide this as good news for Mrs Smothers, perhaps along with the article from Australia.

Where to find the best evidence on interventions

For a woman of her age, Mrs Smothers has a higher risk of experiencing a cardiac event in the coming years than women without her risk factors. It might seem that we already have the evidence to proceed – indeed, an imperative to intervene. But she has asked us to provide evidence that our interventions will help, and rightly so. The intervention question we posed was: In patients like her, does "tight" or "intensive" control of glucose, blood pressure, cholesterol, and proteinuria reduce subsequent morbidity and mortality?

Using the 6S approach, we began with a simple search in MacPLUS FS (http://plus.mcmaster.ca/macplusfs/Default.aspx), a "federated" search engine that simultaneously searches multiple evidence-based resources. As a result, it will most often be a premier resource for one-stop shopping. Alternatives would be to go to Ovid's *Evidence-Based Medicine Reviews*, which also integrates several evidence services, or go directly to a resource that you know to be evidence-based and that you have reason to believe will have an up-to-date version of the information you seek.

Step 2B. Executing the search strategy

Using MacPLUS within our university environment[‡] (which has licensed access to several evidence-based texts and many journals), a search on "diabetes and cardiovascular risk" retrieves information from all levels of the 6S pyramid, except *Systems* (which would require integration of research-based evidence and individual patient information within an electronic medical record – an EMR is available at our institution, but integration with evidence-based guidelines for care is limited to say the least).

[‡]Either by being physically at a computer plugged into the university intranet; or by using "Libaccess", an internet tool that the library provides to authenticate your right to access their licenses online resources, or by "Remote Access" to a university office computer.

At the *Summaries* level (presented in alphabetical order by publication title):

Clinical Evidence (CE; http://clinicalevidence.bmj.com). The first retrieval link from our search leads directly to a one-screen "report card" in *Clinical Evidence* that documents "clear evidence" that cardiovascular outcomes can be reduced in patients with type 2 diabetes through lipid lowering with statins and blood pressure lowering with antihypertensive drugs, and "less well established" evidence that smoking cessation and blood glucose lowering are beneficial. In their narrative, "Intensive glycaemic control and conventional glycaemic control are equally effective at reducing the occurrence of a myocardial infarction, or stroke at 5 years in people with type 2 diabetes and no diagnosis of cardiovascular disease (high-quality evidence)." The text goes on to add: "We don't know whether an intensive insulin treatment with a stepped plan to achieve near normal blood sugar levels is more effective than standard once daily insulin injection at preventing the occurrence of new cardiovascular events in people with type 2 diabetes and previous cardiovascular events (low-quality evidence)." These statements are based on systematic reviews conducted by CE information specialists and authors, and appear to reflect the state of evidence, with one key caveat: the searches were conducted 5 years ago (as of the date of preparation of this chapter), so need checking for more recent evidence. Fortunately, CE provides newer studies for each topic via "Update" tabs and continuously updated searches, and we can look there for newer evidence, so we might not need to look any further than CE for our clinical problem. But let's see what other resources at the *Summaries* level have to offer.

Dynamed (www.ebscohost.com/dynamed). Dynamed presents its information in point form, with levels of evidence (www.ebscohost.com/dynamed/levels.php), and current recommendations from various professional organizations and agencies. For our search, its key points agree with the evidence summaries in *Clinical Evidence* (and the other *Summaries*), e.g., "guidelines generally recommend HbA_{1c} goal of <7% (grade B recommendation [inconsistent or limited evidence]) but note goals should be individualized." Dynamed provides additional emphasis of the potential harms, for example, "target HbA_{1c} <6–6.5% may be more harmful than beneficial (grade B recommendation [inconsistent or limited evidence])". Key recent studies are cited, including ACCORD[10], ADVANCE[11], and VADT[12], but not "in line" with specific recommendations; rather, they appear in a discourse at the end of the section on type 2 diabetes. This is a limitation for anyone who wishes to directly examine the evidence in support of a specific recommendation, observation or level of evidence.

Physicians' Information and Education Resource (PIER; http://pier. acponline.org/index.html or via STAT!Ref). PIER's chapter on type 2 diabetes was recently updated (30 June 2009, just days before our search). Its recommendations are similar to those from *Clinical Evidence*, but it offers these important cautions: "There is some evidence that intensive glucose-lowering treatment aimed at normalizing blood glucose (HbA$_{1c}$ 6%) may be detrimental, at least in middle-aged and older adults with vascular disease or multiple risk factors for vascular disease." The topic review goes on to describe the large ACCORD and ADVANCE trials, published in 2008, and concludes: "Thus, it may now be prudent to target HbA$_{1c}$ to approximately 7% in high-risk patients with type 2 diabetes and multiple risk factors and/or heart disease, especially if aggressive drug therapy is being considered."

UpToDate (www.uptodate.com). *UpToDate*'s summary on this topic was prepared in February 2009 and also summarizes these recent trials, along with the VADT trial. It advises: "… most randomized clinical trials have not demonstrated a beneficial effect of intensive therapy on macrovascular outcomes in type 2 diabetes."

Searching note: It took about 10 minutes to review these three summary resources and the results appear to be consistently impressive from an evidence-based perspective; certainly better than was available when we prepared the third edition of this book 5 years ago. If would be reasonable to stop the search at this point, and apply the findings in decisions with Mrs Smothers. However, it will be instructive to continue the 6S search to see whether additional information is available from the lower levels of the evidence pyramid.

Synopses of syntheses

Selected systematic reviews are provided in synoptic form in *DARE* (which has "open access" at its home base and subscriber access via the Cochrane Library) and in evidence-based journals by subscription. Our search had several hits in these resources, generally supporting the recommendations in the *Summaries*, with some additional information. One of these, a meta-analysis by Selvin and colleagues,[13] assessed the evidence concerning reduction of cardiovascular outcomes with oral antidiabetic medications and concluded that metformin is beneficial while rosiglitazone is possibly harmful, although the evidence for the latter is not strong enough to be conclusive. *DARE* points out some methodologic concerns with the Selvin review but allows that its conclusions are "still likely to be reliable".

A recent synopsis of a synthesis[14] in *ACP Journal Club*[15] concluded that "Metformin did not improve a composite of microvascular and macrovascular disease but reduced macrovascular disease, prevented weight gain, and improved glycemic control with less insulin in patients with type 2 diabetes." Thus, we'll want to continue metformin in Mrs Smothers' regimen, if she is tolerating it and willing to take it.

Another, even more recent, *ACPJC* synopsis[16] of a synthesis by Ray et al.,[17] shows that 131 patients with type 2 diabetes would need to be treated for 5 years to reduce one non-fatal myocardial infarction, with no evidence of a decrease in overall mortality, but with increased risk for serious hypoglycemia and congestive heart failure (possibly associated with glitazone use).

Syntheses

Again our search is rewarding at the *Syntheses* level. For example, a review,[18] published 2 weeks before this chapter was written (and available through *EvidenceUpdates, ACPJC+,* and *MacPLUS*) summarized the evidence concerning lipid lowering in people without CVS disease but with CVS risk factors, and documents "significantly improved survival and large reductions in the risk of major cardiovascular events", including for people with diabetes.

An earlier review[19] summarizes the benefits of "tight" blood pressure control for patients with type 2 diabetes, providing 10-year "numbers needed to treat" (NNTs – see Chapter 5 for definitions) of nine for preventing any diabetes outcome and 24 for preventing all cause mortality.

There is also supplementary information on the effect of weight-loss drugs for type 2 diabetes[20] (short-term improvement in glycemic control; long-term, patient-important benefits and adverse effects not known). Thus, our management of Mrs Smothers' diabetes will need to be to attend to the incomplete control of her hypertension and dyslipidemia.

Synopses of studies

Individual studies of high quality and clinical relevance are synopsized in the evidence-based journals and provide some additional information of value for our management of Mrs Smothers. For example, the impressive study of Gaede and colleagues[21] is abstracted in *ACP Journal Club,* showing the long-term morbidity and mortality benefits of multiple cardiovascular risk factor intervention for patients with type 2 diabetes and microproteinuria. Many of the original studies that were summarized, synthesized and synopsized at higher levels of the evidence hierarchy are here for inspection, for example, to determine who was studied in relation to our patient, Mrs Smothers. It does appear that she is similar to the patients included in the Gaede study, which is good news for her, as the study specifically addresses the benefits of multiple risk factor intervention.

Studies

This lowest level of the 6S pyramid is large and less wieldy, requiring more sorting and appraisal by the user. It is worth noting that it takes time for studies to be digested by the higher levels of the pyramid, and this can take weeks to months to years, depending on the service. In most cases, new studies will not provide a strong enough discordant signal to change the message of the syntheses and summaries at higher levels, but new "landmark" studies can be published at any time, and non-landmark studies can also attract a lot of press coverage, with patients as their primary audience. Thus, it is helpful to practitioners to be able to access current studies, and our search includes them.

The studies are at three levels – in descending order of clinical usefulness: (1) pre-appraised for quality and relevance (e.g., via *ACPJC+* and *EvidenceUpdates*); (2) retrieved via clinical queries from MEDLINE; and (3) retrieved via PubMed using just our search terms, "type 2 diabetes and cardiovascular risk". As you can imagine, the number of articles retrieved increases dramatically at the lowest levels and the amount of appraisal you will need to do increases accordingly. Nevertheless, it is easy to discard many of the articles just on the basis of their titles, and some heavy lifting will often yield a few nuggets. Examples that might be of interest in this case include studies of: low glycemic-index diet vs high-fiber cereal diet[22] (low glycemic-index diet improved glycemic control over 6 months), endurance vs strength training and their combination[23] (the combo worked best for glycemic control and CVS risk), and a comparison of the UKPDS risk engine vs Framingham[9] (UKPDS worked better than Framingham but considerably overestimated cardiac risk in a contemporary Australian cohort of people with type 2 diabetes), which we also found at a higher level of the pyramid.

What about traditional textbooks of medicine?

If you don't use traditional medical texts, you've already correctly answered this question. If you do use traditional texts in print or online, please check to see if they provide the detailed, up-to-date, evidential basis for care that we've just surveyed. Send us the name of any text that you feel merits a score of 6 or more (passing grade) on the 11-point scale in Table 2.1. Any that don't should not be used to support healthcare decisions, although they might be brilliant for "background" information.

Step 2C. Examining the evidence

We've quickly assembled the summary, synopsis, and study level pre-appraised information needed to inform evidence-based decisions for Mrs Smothers. Her diabetes, blood pressure, and lipids are not well controlled, she is overweight and she continues to smoke. She is worried about cardiovascular consequences, given her sister's premature demise, and her UKPDS risk score is high, but that may be overestimating her actual risk, especially if her risk factors are lowered. Key recent studies, ACCORD,[10] ADVANCE,[11] VADT,[12] show little or no macrovascular benefit of intensive control for type 2 diabetes, and increased risk for severe hypoglycemia, but the long-term follow-up of UKPDS participants documents the benefits of not-quite-so-intensive control of diabetes. The Gaede et al.[21] Steno2 report documents the substantial benefits of multiple risk factor intervention for type 2 diabetes, including both macrovascular (cardiac and cerebrovascular) and microvascular (diabetic nephropathy, retinopathy, and neuropathy) outcomes. Smoking cessation is important for so many adverse events that it needs to be included on the list of management priorities. Weight reduction, including the use of medications to achieve it, would have at least short-term benefits, so needs to be taken into account, although not with the same imperative as the other interventions.

Thus, the list of targets for which validated, beneficial interventions can be offered includes dyslipidemia, high blood pressure, hyperglycemia and smoking. Should she decide to deal with her smoking, the 6S pyramid is well populated by validated interventions, from the summaries level on down. The easiest-to-implement-high-payoff interventions, however, are likely to be a daily statin and ACE-inhibitor, and encouragement to take all prescribed doses of her metformin.

Practice makes perfect

For further practice in finding the best evidence, you might want to tackle the question of whether vitamin E and beta-carotene are Mrs Smothers' friends, foes, or just fees for her.

Step 1. Asking an answerable question

In high cardiovascular risk smokers, do vitamin E and beta-carotene prevent clinical events or death, compared with not taking these chemicals?

Step 2A–C. Selecting an evidence resource; executing the search strategy; examining the evidence

A quick search (5 seconds) of *MacPLUS* for "antioxidants and cardiovascular risk" retrieved items from the *Summaries* level down, including a synopsis of a recent Cochrane systematic review of large trials of antioxidant vitamins, vitamin E or beta-carotene, for the primary or secondary prevention of mortality or cardiovascular disease.[24] No benefits were found among the 232 550 participants of 67 RCTs. Worse still, a second review reported that beta-carotene supplements increase mortality from cancer among smokers.[25]

With all this evidence showing no benefit of antioxidants, you wonder what the hype on them is about – and why beta-carotene is still available in pharmacies over-the-counter, alone and as a common constituent of multivitamins. Should you post a warning on the wall of your clinic?

Just for practice, try your hand with PubMed (www.ncbi.nlm.nih.gov/PubMed/) and PubMed Clinical Queries (www.ncbi.nlm.nih.gov/entrez/query/static/clinical.html). A search on beta-carotene or vitamin E using PubMed (in July 2009) retrieved 37 067 references! Although most of them have something to do with the general topic, we gave up when the first 20 citations did not appear to address our question directly (most had to do with rats and test tubes). Searches in such a large database require more exacting search techniques. Switching to PubMed's Clinical Queries, selecting the Systematic Reviews option, and using the same search terms plus "and cardiovascular" retrieves 53 citations including several apparently pertinent reviews, the Cochrane review[24] among them (in 11th position).

Applying the evidence

Evidence can build a strong foundation for helping Mrs Smothers with her problems, including gaining an accurate prognosis, determining current best methods for reducing her risks for adverse cardiovascular and diabetes outcomes, and providing her with information concerning non-prescribed treatments she is taking. However, it is important to observe that "evidence does not make decisions".[3] Other key components are her clinical circumstances and her wishes. It is important to note that her circumstances include a number of medical problems: poorly controlled diabetes, hypertension, dyslipidemia, obesity, and smoking. Dealing with all these problems simultaneously is unlikely to occur because of the heavy behavioral demands of the complex regimen that would be required to treat them all successfully. (If you doubt this for an instant, try following the "ideal prescription" that you would prescribe for Mrs Smothers, substituting candies for pills, and "low-glycemic index" foods if you don't have her conditions. Our prediction: you won't make it through a day without failing on one or more of your instructions.) Furthermore, she indicates suboptimal adherence (she does not always take her metformin, an admission that is associated with less than 50% adherence[26]).

You will need to carefully negotiate priorities with the patient to find the best match between the evidence and her wishes, then incorporate current best evidence concerning interventions to help her follow the treatments that she has agreed to accept.[27] Thus, the evidence you have accumulated in this chapter will get you only part of the way towards the decisions that Mrs Smothers and you will need to make, but at least your decisions will be informed by the best available evidence concerning her risks and the interventions that will reduce or, in the case of beta-carotene, increase them. We'll discuss the application of evidence about therapy in further detail in Chapter 5.

Other ways to find evidence

The *MacPLUS* search engine provides a focussed approach to tracking down evidence for clinical decisions that will serve well for many clinical problems, but it is currently under development and testing. We expect it will be widely available before this book is published, but can't guarantee it. A fallback would be getting to know each of the resources PLUS searches and selecting the appropriate resources to search one at a time for the question(s) you are addressing. For example, if the question is one of diagnosis, *UpToDate* could work, but *Clinical Evidence* would not, since it doesn't include diagnostic evidence. Similarly, the Cochrane Library does not include many diagnostic reviews at present, but they are beginning to increase in numbers.

If you don't know exactly where to look first, TRIP and SUMSearch, described earlier in this chapter, provide the most general search engines for evidence-based content.

Don't forget to subscribe to a "push" publication that suits your needs and allows you to tailor alerts to your area(s) of clinical interest.

References

1. Pickering GW. The purpose of medical education. *BMJ*. 1956;2:113–116.

2. DiCenso A, Bayley E, Haynes RB. Accessing pre-appraised evidence: fine-tuning the 5S model into a 6S model. *Evid Based Nurs*. 2009;12(4):99–101.

3. Haynes RB, Devereaux PJ, Guyatt GH. Clinical expertise in the era of evidence-based medicine and patient choice. *ACP J Club*. 2002; 136(2):A11–A13.

4. Garg AX, Adhikari N, McDonald H, et al. Effects of computerized clinical decision support systems on practitioner performance and patient outcomes: a systematic review. *JAMA*. 2005;293(10):1323–1338.

5. Manns B, ACP J Club. Review: Brand-name drugs are not more effective than generic versions for treating cardiovascular disease. [Abstract for Kesselheim AS, Misono AS, Lee JL, et al. Clinical equivalence of generic and brand-name drugs used in cardiovascular disease: a systematic review and meta-analysis. *JAMA*. 2008;300(21):2514–2526.] *Ann Intern Med*. 2009;150(8):JC4–JC6.

6. McKibbon KA, Wilczynski NL, Haynes RB. What do evidence-based secondary journals tell us about the publication of clinically important articles in primary healthcare journals? *BMC Med*. 2004;2:33.

7. Bruce SA. Review: inhaled corticosteroids do not reduce mortality but increase pneumonia in chronic obstructive pulmonary disease. *Evid Based Nurs*. 2009;12(3):76.

8. Stevens RJ, Kothari V, Adler AI, et al. United Kingdom Prospective Diabetes Study (UKPDS) Group. The UKPDS risk engine: a model for the risk of coronary heart disease in type II diabetes (UKPDS 56). *Clin Sci (Lond)*. 2001;101:671–679.

9. Colagiuri DWA, Davis TMS. Comparison of the Framingham and United Kingdom Prospective Diabetes Study cardiovascular risk equations in Australian patients with type 2 diabetes from the Fremantle Diabetes Study. *Med J Aust*. 2009;190:180–184.

10. Gerstein HC, Miller ME, Byington RP, et al. Action to Control Cardiovascular Risk in Diabetes Study Group. Effects of intensive glucose lowering in type 2 diabetes. *N Engl J Med*. 2008;358(24):2545–2559.

11. Patel A, MacMahon S, Chalmers J, et al. ADVANCE Collaborative Group. Intensive blood glucose control and vascular outcomes in patients with type 2 diabetes. *N Engl J Med.* 2008;358(24):2560–2572.

12. Duckworth W, Abraira C, Moritz T, et al. Glucose control and vascular complications in veterans with type 2 diabetes. *N Engl J Med.* 2009;360(2):129–139.

13. Selvin E, Bolen S, Yeh HC, et al. Cardiovascular outcomes in trials of oral diabetes medications: a systematic review. *Arch Intern Med.* 2008;168(19):2070–2080.

14. Kooy A, de Jager J, Lehert P, et al. Long-term effects of metformin on metabolism and microvascular and macrovascular disease in patients with type 2 diabetes mellitus. *Arch Intern Med.* 2009;169(6):616–625.

15. Fonseca V, ACP J Club. Adding metformin to insulin did not improve a composite of microvascular and macrovascular disease in type 2 diabetes. *Ann Intern Med.* 2009;151(2):JC1–JC12.

16. Lipscombe LL, ACP J Club. Review: Intensive glucose control reduced some CV events but did not change mortality in type 2 diabetes. *Ann Intern Med.* 2009;151(6):JC3–JC6.

17. Ray KK, Seshasai SR, Wijesuriya S, et al. Effect of intensive control of glucose on cardiovascular outcomes and death in patients with diabetes mellitus: a meta-analysis of randomised controlled trials. *Lancet.* 2009;373(9677):1765–1772.

18. Brugts JJ, Yetgin T, Hoeks SE, et al. The benefits of statins in people without established cardiovascular disease but with cardiovascular risk factors: meta-analysis of randomised controlled trials. *BMJ.* 2009;338:b2376.

19. Vijan S, Hayward RA. Treatment of hypertension in type 2 diabetes mellitus: blood pressure goals, choice of agents, and setting priorities in diabetes care. *Ann Intern Med.* 2003;138(7):593–602.

20. Lloret-Linares C, Greenfield JR, Czernichow S. Effect of weight-reducing agents on glycaemic parameters and progression to Type 2 diabetes: a review. *Diabet Med.* 2008;25(10):1142–1150.

21. Gaede P, Lund-Andersen H, Parving HH, et al. Effect of a multifactorial intervention on mortality in type 2 diabetes. *N Engl J Med.* 2008;358(6):580–591.

22. Jenkins DJ, Kendall CW, McKeown-Eyssen G, et al. Effect of a low-glycemic index or a high-cereal fiber diet on type 2 diabetes: a randomized trial. *JAMA.* 2008;300(23):2742–2753.

23. Lambers S, Van Laethem C, Van Acker K, et al. Influence of combined exercise training on indices of obesity, diabetes and cardiovascular risk in type 2 diabetes patients. *Clin Rehabil.* 2008;22(6):483–492.

2

24. Bjelakovic G, Nikolova D, Gluud L, et al. Antioxidant supplements for prevention of mortality in healthy participants and patients with various diseases. *Cochrane Database Syst Rev.* 2008;(2) CD007176.

25. Vivekananthan DP, Penn MS, Sapp SK, et al. Use of antioxidant vitamins for the prevention of cardiovascular disease: meta-analysis of randomised trials. *Lancet.* 2003;361(9374):2017–2023.

26. Stephenson BJ, Rowe BH, Macharia WM, et al. The rational clinical examination. Is this patient taking the treatment as prescribed? *JAMA.* 1993;269(21):2779–2781.

27. Tierney WM. Review: Evidence on the effectiveness of interventions to assist patient adherence to prescribed medications is limited. [Abstract for McDonald HP, Garg AX, Haynes RB. Interventions to enhance patient adherence to medication prescriptions: scientific review. *JAMA.* 2002;288(22):2868–2879.] *ACP J Club.* 2002;139(1):19.

3 Appraising the evidence

We've finished our literature search and we've identified some evidence. Now we need to decide if it's valid and important before we can apply the evidence to our individual patients. The order in which we consider validity and importance depends on individual preference. We could start by appraising its validity arguing that if it isn't valid, who cares whether it appears to show a huge effect? Alternatively, we could determine its clinical importance arguing that if the evidence doesn't suggest a clinically important impact, who cares if it's valid? We can start with either question, as long as we remember to follow-up one favorable answer with the other question.

There are many sources of potential bias (defined as the systematic deviation from the truth) which can affect the validity of studies and thus affect whether we believe their results. We're not going to describe all of the potential sources of bias here (we refer you to some classic readings at the end of this section). Instead, in subsequent chapters, we'll address some of the key sources of bias in different study types that we need to consider in order to become effective consumers of the literature.

There are some features common to appraisal of most studies of therapy, diagnosis, prognosis, and etiology/harm. Paul Glasziou has suggested we consider a race analogy to illustrate these commonalities. First, was there a fair start? This would include consideration of what is the population of interest? How were they identified? Was the population appropriately selected? Was assignment to the intervention or exposure appropriate? Second, was the race fair? Specifically, were the study participants treated the same throughout? Did they all complete the study? Third, was it a fair finish? Was there an appropriate measurement of outcomes, namely blind and/or objective? Was the analysis of results appropriate? We'll review these concepts in more detail in subsequent chapters.

Note that rather than the racing analogy, we could use the PICO format when we consider validity. First, what is the population/who are the patients, requires consideration of how were they recruited and whether it is an appropriate target population. Second, what was the intervention, exposure, test that they experienced and how was this exposure/treatment/test allocated? Third, were outcomes measured in a blind and/or objective fashion; and, when were they measured? We'll discuss each of these issues (and potential sources of bias) in subsequent chapters.

As mentioned in Chapter 2, when we're performing a literature search we should seek an overview that systematically searches for and combines evidence from all studies relevant to the topic because this will provide us with a more reliable answer to our clinical question than the results from a single study. Systematic reviews of the literature are most commonly found for therapy topics and we'll review them in detail in Chapter 4. However, we are starting to see more systematic reviews of prognosis, diagnostic test accuracy and harm and there are validity concerns common to all of these systematic reviews. Namely:

1. Was the literature search comprehensive? This question includes consideration of whether the authors included studies from appropriate electronic databases; did they use additional sources for identifying studies such as hand-searching journals or contacting experts in the field; and, did the authors place any language restrictions on their search results?

2. Was the quality of the individual studies assessed? We would like to see that the investigators critically appraised the individual studies for validity (using criteria similar to those which we describe in subsequent chapters) and that they provided an explicit methodology for this.

In subsequent chapters, following discussion of the validity of the studies (whether individual studies or systematic reviews) we'll consider whether its results are important. This discussion will include a consideration of the magnitude and precision of the results. For systematic reviews, we also want to consider heterogeneity – whether the results are consistent from study to study.

There are many different critical appraisal worksheets and checklists that can be used when considering validity of individual studies. While we provide one format in this book, on the accompanying CD we provide examples of others that you might want to review, including the GATE assessment tool which has been developed by Rod Jackson. There is no one single way of critically appraising a study or of teaching critical appraisal (indeed, we're only limited by our imaginations!) and we encourage you to find strategies that work for you and your learners.

For now, sit back, relax and let's see how the race to the finish unfolds!

Further reading

Guyatt G, Rennie D, Meade M, et al., eds. *Users' guides to the medical literature. A manual for evidence-based clinical practice*. Chicago: AMA Press; 2008.

Haynes RB, Sackett DL, Guyatt GH, et al. *Clinical epidemiology: How to do clinical practice research*. Philadelphia: Lippincott Williams & Wilkins; 2006.

Sackett DL. Bias in analytic research. *J Chronic Dis*. 1979;32(1–2):51–63.

3

4 Therapy

In this chapter, we're going to tackle the critical appraisal of therapy articles. We'll start by considering individual trials. To illustrate our discussion, we'll consider the following scenario.

Clinical scenario

We have in our practice a 76-year-old man who was admitted to a long-term care facility 1 year ago. He has a history of Alzheimer disease and was admitted because his family could no longer provide care for him at home due to his agitation and wandering. His daughter is also in our practice and we have chatted with her on many occasions about admitting her father to long-term care, which was a difficult decision for her to make. She is her father's substitute decision-maker for personal care. Her father was started on antipsychotics to help manage his behavior. She wonders if these medications will decrease his agitation and she's particularly concerned about potential adverse effects because she read recently on the internet that antipsychotics may cause harm. She knows that her father has been on risperidone and haloperidol for more than 1 year. Currently he receives risperidone 1 mg twice daily and occasionally receives a PRN dose of haloperidol. He has stable angina and is otherwise well.

Based on this scenario, we posed the following question, "In a patient with a history of Alzheimer disease and agitation, does therapy with antipsychotics such as risperidone and haloperidol decrease the risk of agitation and increase the risk of death?" Using PubMed Clinical Queries (see Ch. 2 for a description of this search engine) and the search terms "dementia" and "antipsychotics", we identified a recent trial[1] which might help us answer this question. This trial specifically addresses the impact of these medications on mortality but also refers to another trial which provides some information on impact on behavior. (We also found this first trial in *ACP Journal Club*).[2] Note that this is a question that requires consideration of benefits and harms of a potential therapy. There is always good and bad with everything in life, including potential therapeutic interventions.

Types of therapeutic reports

In this Chapter, we will initially tackle how to assess evidence about therapy from individual studies. However, individual trials (unless it's a large, high-quality randomized trial) are not the best evidence that we can find about the effects of therapy, and ideally, we should seek a systematic review. Guides for determining their validity are in Table 4.1. However, because systematic reviews assess their component trials individually (and because we want to be sure that they've done so in a valid way), and since at this point in time we're still more likely to find individual trials than systematic reviews, we'll begin with discussing the individual trial. Sometimes the trial(s) will be insufficient by themselves for decision-making and extrapolation or a detailed examination of the tradeoffs between the benefits and harms of the intervention might be warranted and our literature search might be extended to find a clinical decision analysis. Rules for deciding whether it's valid are presented in Table 4.15. Similarly, we may want to track down an economic analysis, and questions that will help us decide whether we can believe the results are listed in Table 4.18. Clinical practice guidelines outline evidence about diagnosis, prognosis and therapy for a particular target disorder and guides for helping us decide if we want to apply them are in Table 4.21. Qualitative studies can sometimes help guide us in our therapeutic decision-making, and criteria to help us consider their validity are in Table 4.14. Finally, we may not be able to track down evidence that clearly helps us and our patients when making a decision about therapy and in these cases, we might want to consider completing an "N-of-1" study (Table 4.25).

CARDS

Table 4.1 Is this evidence about therapy (from an individual randomized trial) valid?

Was there a fair start?
1. Was the assignment of patients to treatment randomized?
2. Was the randomization concealed?
3. Were the groups similar at the start of the trial?

Was there a fair race?
4. Was follow-up of patients sufficiently long and complete?
5. Were all patients analyzed in the groups to which they were randomized?

Some finer points:
6. Were patients, clinicians and study personnel kept blind to treatment?
7. Were groups treated equally, apart from the experimental therapy?

Reports of individual studies

Are the results of this individual study valid?

See Table 4.1.

1. Was the assignment of patients to treatment randomized?

Until recently, it was believed that hormone replacement therapy (HRT) could decrease the risk of coronary artery disease (CAD) in post-menopausal women with a history of established CAD. This belief was based on data from several observational studies that found women who used HRT had a decreased risk of the disease.[3] Clinicians and patients were subsequently surprised by the results of a randomized trial of women with established CAD, which found that the risk of CAD was not reduced with HRT.[4] More recently, the Women's Health Initiative study found that HRT was not effective in the primary prevention of CAD either.[5]

There are lots of examples where the completion of randomized trials has yielded surprising results, in contrast with that found in observational studies or from results hypothesized from "first principles". For example, case series and case reports of extracranial–intracranial (EC/IC) arterial bypass suggested benefit from this surgery, but a randomized trial of EC/IC bypass compared with medical treatment alone found no benefit from surgery.[6] Ventricular arrhythmias in patients who had a myocardial infarction were found to be a risk factor for death. It was thought that if these arrhythmias were suppressed (with agents such as encainide and flecainide), mortality would be decreased in these patients. However, results from a randomized trial (CAST) found more harm than good resulted from these agents.[7] Indeed, it has been estimated that more Americans died from receiving these agents than from the Vietnam War in the same time period.[8]

Why such a difference between the results of the observational studies and the randomized trials? In observational studies, the patient's and/or clinician's preferences determine whether or not the patient receives the treatment. Often, factors such as the presence of co-morbid illnesses, use of other medications, the individual's beliefs, and the severity of the disease and its symptoms, influence the patient's and physician's therapeutic decision-making process and these same factors can also influence the risk of the outcome of interest (e.g., CAD).

If these prognostic factors are unevenly distributed between treatment groups, this could exaggerate, cancel or even counteract the effects of therapy.*

Randomization balances the treatment groups for prognostic factors, even if we don't yet know enough about the target disorder to know what they all are. If these factors exaggerated the apparent effects of an otherwise ineffectual treatment, the effects of their imbalance could lead to the false-positive conclusion that the treatment was useful when in fact it wasn't. In contrast, if they nullified or counteracted the effects of a really efficacious treatment, this could lead to a false-negative conclusion that a useful treatment was useless or even harmful. We should insist on random allocation to treatment because it comes closer than any other research design to creating groups of patients at the start of the trial who are identical in their risk of the event we are trying to prevent. We need to determine if the investigators used some method analogous to tossing a coin† to assign patients to treatment groups (e.g., the experimental treatment is assigned if the coin landed "heads" and a conventional, "control" or "placebo"‡ treatment is given if the coin landed "tails").

Randomization is something for investigators to be proud of and often you'll find it mentioned explicitly in the abstract (or the title). If the study wasn't randomized, we'd suggest that you stop reading it and go on to the next article in your search. *(Note: We can begin to rapidly critically appraise article literature by scanning the abstract to determine if the study is randomized, if it isn't we can bin it.)* Only if you can't find any randomized trials should you go back to it. If, however, the sole evidence you have about a treatment is from non-randomized studies, you have five options:

1. Check Chapter 2 again or get some help in doing another literature search to see if you missed any randomized trials of the therapy.

2. Assess whether the treatment effect described in the non-randomized trial is so huge that you can't imagine it could be a

---

*Patient characteristics that are extraneous to the question posed, could cause the clinical outcome that we are trying to prevent with the treatment, and might be unevenly distributed between the treatment groups, are called confounders. Although there are other easy ways to avoid confounding (exclusion, stratified sampling, matching, stratified analysis, standardization and multivariate modeling), they all require that we already know what the confounder is.

†In practice, this should be done by computers but the principle remains the same.

‡A placebo is a treatment that is so similar in appearance, taste, etc. to the active treatment, that the patient, clinician and study personnel cannot distinguish it.

false-positive study (this is very rare, and usually only satisfied when the prognosis of untreated patients is uniformly terrible, such as everyone with bacterial meningitis dying prior to the use of antibiotics). As a check, you could ask your colleagues whether they consider the candidate therapy so likely to be efficacious that they'd consider it unethical to randomize a patient like your's into a study that includes a no-treatment or placebo group.

3. If the non-randomized trial concluded that the treatment was useless or harmful, then it is usually safe to accept that conclusion. False-positive conclusions from non-randomized studies are far more common than false-negative ones (e.g., since treatments are typically withheld from patients with the poorest prognoses, and patients who faithfully take their medicine are destined for better outcomes, even when they are taking worthless treatments or placebos!).

4. Consider whether an "N-of-1" trial would make sense to you and your patient. These are useful in chronic disease management (Table 4.25).

5. Try to find evidence for another management option.

In the trial that we found, by Ballard and colleagues,[1] to answer our question about antipsychotic therapy, the title states that it is a randomized trial and a quick scan of the methods reveals a description of randomization. Patients were randomized to either continue treatment for 12 months or be switched to a placebo. Our study mentions that randomization included a minimization algorithm. Minimization is a strategy used to achieve balance in prognostic factors. It is particularly useful in small trials. Typically, we'd begin by identifying the prognostic factors we want balanced. Then we would dichotomize them at a clinically sensible point. In our study, the investigators used the following prognostic factors: a Mini Mental State Examination score of <6; presence or absence of extrapyramidal signs, visual hallucinations and delusions; use of cholinesterase inhibitors; and current use of antipsychotic medications. If the first recruited patient has an MMSE of 5, is on cholinesterase inhibitors and antipsychotic medications, he'd be allocated a score of 3. Using the computerized randomization process, he is randomized to the intervention group. The next patient has a score of 1 (for use of cholinesterase inhibitors) and to minimize the difference in total scores between the intervention and control groups, he is allocated to the control group.

2. Was the randomization concealed?

Was randomization concealed from the clinicians and study personnel who entered patients into the trial? If allocation was concealed, the clinicians would be unaware of which treatment the next patient would receive and thus unable, consciously or unconsciously, to distort the balance between the groups being compared. Knowledge of the next assignment could lead to the exclusion of certain patients based on their prognosis because they would have been allocated to the perceived inappropriate group. As with failure to use randomization, inadequate concealment of allocation can distort the apparent effect of treatment in either direction, causing the effect to seem larger or smaller than it really is. Often, articles don't state whether the randomization list was concealed, but if randomization occurred by telephone or by some system that was at a distance from where patients were being entered into the trial, we can be assured by this.

It has been shown that investigators report overcoming virtually every type of allocation concealment strategy – from holding an envelope to a bright light, to ransacking office files of the principal investigator to find the allocation list![9] (Allocation concealment will not be achieved by using transparent envelopes – even if they're sealed!) Ideally, we'd like to see randomization being done centrally, by computer, at a distance from where allocation is occurring. Assignments should be received one at a time, as each patient is enrolled to prevent receiving a number of assignments at once – which could lead to disruption in randomization.

> In the study we found, randomization was done centrally at a location remote from where patients were enrolled. The statistician who did the randomization had no direct contact with patients.

3. Were the groups similar at the start of the trial?

We should check to see if the groups were similar in all prognostically important ways (except for receiving the treatment) at the start of the trial. As noted above, the benefit of randomization is the equal distribution of potential confounders between the study groups. However, baseline differences between the study groups may be present due to chance. There is usually no value to providing p values in the table describing baseline characteristics of participants. These hypotheses tests assess the probability that differences observed could be due to chance. In well-designed randomized trials, any observed differences are due to chance. Studies have shown that researchers who use hypothesis tests to compare baseline characteristics report fewer significant results than expected by chance.[8] This might be because investigators may not report significant differences in baseline characteristics because of concern that this might impact credibility of their results. If the groups aren't similar, we must determine if adjustment for these potentially important prognostic factors was carried out. It is reassuring if the adjusted and un-adjusted analyses yield similar results.

> In the antipsychotics study, a scan of Table 4.1 in the paper reveals that there were no important differences between patients in the two groups.

4. Was follow-up of patients sufficiently long and complete?

Once we are satisfied that the study was randomized, we can look to see if all patients who were entered into the trial were accounted for at its conclusion. Determining this has become easier with the inclusion of flow diagrams (Figure 4.1) in the trial that we found. Inclusion of a flow diagram is part of the CONSORT statement, which aims to enhance reporting accuracy of trials.[10] Many journals have adopted this statement and this has made it easier to review articles for validity.

Ideally, we'd like to see that no patients were lost to follow-up because these patients may have had outcomes that would affect the conclusions of the study. If, for example, patients receiving the experimental treatment dropped out because of adverse outcomes, their absence from the analysis would lead to an overestimation of the efficacy of the treatment (and underreporting of potential adverse events from the intervention).

What can we consider to be an acceptable loss? To be sure of a trial's conclusion, the investigators should be able to take all patients who were lost to follow-up, assign them the worst case outcome (assume that everyone lost from the group whose remaining members fared better had a bad outcome and assume that everyone lost from the group whose remaining members fared worse had a good outcome), and still be able to support their original conclusion. If this method doesn't change the study's conclusions, the loss to follow-up is not a threat to the study's validity. However, if the study

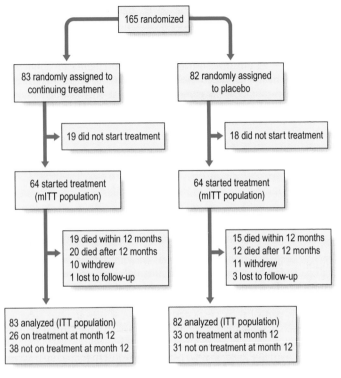

Figure 4.1 CONSORT diagram.[1]

result does change, its validity is threatened and we must decide if the results derived from the worst case method are plausible. It would be unusual for a trial to withstand a worst case analysis if it lost more than 20% of its patients (but this depends on the number of outcomes observed, for example, if few outcomes were observed in a large study, the loss of 20% of patients could have a big impact on the results) and journals like *ACP Journal Club* won't publish trials with a less than 80% follow-up.

We should also ensure that the follow-up of patients was sufficiently long to see a clinically important effect. For example, if our study assessing the use of antipsychotics and risk of death only followed patients for 1 week or 1 month, we wouldn't find the results very helpful. Given the nature of the target disorder, we'd like to see a follow-up period of several months or, ideally, years. One of the challenges that we face as clinicians is that often drugs are used for longer periods of time than in studied trials. For example, there is a lack of trials of serotonin reuptake inhibitors lasting more than 1 year for treatment of depression, although these agents are often used for several years.[11] This is an issue we need to consider when deciding on applicability of therapy studies. Finally, we often see trials stopped early when a large benefit is seen. When sample size and number of outcomes are small, this overestimate of the treatment effect can be dangerous and the results of such a study should be interpreted with caution.[12] Sometimes information about follow-up is available in the study's abstract but most often we have to turn to the results to obtain specific details.

In our study, investigators were able to follow-up all patients to 12 months.

5. Were all patients analyzed in the groups to which they were randomized?

Because anything that happens after randomization can affect the chance that a study patient has the outcome of interest, it's important that all patients (even those who fail to take their medicine or accidentally or intentionally receive the wrong treatment) are analyzed in the groups to which they were allocated. Once comparable groups are setup at the study onset, they should stay this way to preserve randomization. It has been shown repeatedly that patients who "do" and "don't" take their study medicine have very different outcomes, even when the study medicine is a placebo. The study participants that left the study or crossed over into another treatment group may have a particular characteristic so that those remaining in the groups are no longer as comparable as they were at the study onset. To preserve the value of randomization, we should demand an "intention-to-treat analysis", whereby all patients are analyzed in the groups to which they were initially assigned, regardless of whether they received their assigned treatment. It is important that we not only look for the term "intention-to-treat analysis" in the methods but also look at the results to ensure that this analysis was actually done.

The antipsychotics study used an intention-to-treat analysis.

6. Were patients, clinicians and study personnel kept blind to treatment?

Blinding is necessary to avoid the patient's reporting of symptoms or their adherence to treatment being affected by hunches about whether the treatment is effective. Similarly, blinding prevents the report or interpretation of symptoms from being affected by the clinician's or outcomes assessor's suspicions about the effectiveness of the study intervention. Not surprisingly, blinding is particularly important when the outcome of interest is subjective and more judgment by the clinician or outcomes assessor is necessary.

When patients and clinicians can't be kept blind (such as in some surgical trials), often it is possible to have other blinded clinicians assess clinical records (purged of any mention of treatment), or to use objective outcome measurements. For example, in the North American Symptomatic Carotid Endarterectomy Trial[13] (this study randomized patients with symptomatic carotid stenosis to either carotid endarterectomy or medical therapy with aspirin), the patients in the surgical group (and the surgeons performing the procedure) could obviously not be blinded to the treatment. Outcome events were assessed by four groups: the participating neurologist and surgeon; the neurologist at the study centre; "blinded" members of the steering committee; and "blinded" external adjudicators.

Clinicians interpret the term "double blind" differently, and ideally an article should explicitly state who was blinded, but it is rare to find articles that do this. Information about blinding may be present in the abstract or the methods section (and sometimes the title) of the article.[14]

> The trial description published in *The Lancet Neurology* states that it was a double-blind placebo-controlled trial. It also mentions that outcomes assessors were blinded. A review of the *ACP Journal Club* abstract of this trial identifies that patients, caregivers and relatives, clinicians, patients administering trial drugs and outcome assessors were blinded; this information was provided by the authors on request from the *ACP Journal Club*.

7. Were groups treated equally, apart from the experimental therapy?

Blinding of patients, clinicians and study personnel can prevent them from adding any additional treatments (or "co-interventions"), apart from the experimental treatment, to just one of the groups. For example, were patients in the intervention group in our study more likely to have received other interventions to address agitation? Usually we can find information about co-interventions in the methods and/or results sections of an article.

If the study fails any of the criteria discussed above, we need to decide if the flaw is significant and threatens the validity of the study. If this is the case, we'll need to look for another study. If we find that our article satisfies all of the criteria, we can proceed to consideration of its importance.

> We believe that our study has satisfied all the major validity criteria and we will look at its results.

> *Note*: How many validity criteria are mentioned in the abstract of the original article? In the study we identified, the abstract mentions randomization, intention to treat analysis and the percentage of patients who were followed. While not all of the validity criteria are mentioned, seeing these in the abstract helps us to assess the article more quickly. We can then move to the Methods section to search for the other validity criteria.

4

Are the valid results of this individual study important?

In this section, we'll discuss how to determine if the potential benefits (or harms) of the treatment described in a study are important. We'll refer to the guides in Table 4.2 for this discussion. Deciding whether we should be impressed with the results of a trial requires two steps: first, finding the most useful clinical expression of these results; and second, comparing these results with the results of other treatments for other target disorders.

1. What is the magnitude of the treatment effect?

Consideration of the magnitude of the results requires assessment of the outcomes that are included in the study. To date we have limited discussion to focus on the outcomes that were relevant to our patient

Table 4.2 Is this valid evidence about therapy (from an individual randomized trial) important?

1. What is the magnitude of the treatment effect?
2. How precise is the estimate of the treatment effect?

77

and his daughter. Sometimes trials will report on surrogate outcomes which refer to outcomes other than those that are important to patients. These outcomes can be acceptable if they are shown to be valid surrogates for clinically important outcomes. For example, in studies assessing the effectiveness of osteoporosis therapy, ideally the trials should include measurement of the impact of the intervention on fractures. However, bone mineral density (BMD) is a surrogate outcome that is often used in these studies. BMD has been shown to correlate with fracture risk and therefore is an acceptable surrogate outcome. Surrogate outcomes are often used because they can reduce sample size and follow-up time.

Composite outcomes are also seen frequently in trials and trials that use them must be assessed cautiously.[15] For example, in the ADVANCE trial, more than 11 000 patients with type 2 diabetes mellitus were randomized to intensive therapy (target A_{1C} of <6.5%) or standard therapy (target A_{1C} >6.5%).[16] The primary outcome was a composite outcome including macrovascular (non-fatal MI or stroke or death from cardiovascular causes) or microvascular events (worsening nephropathy or retinopathy). Worsening nephropathy was defined as macroalbuminuria, doubling of serum creatinine, renal replacement therapy or death from renal causes. A significant difference was seen in the composite outcome of macrovascular and microvascular events (Table 4.3). Teasing these results apart, it is apparent that there was no significant difference in macrovascular events. Microvascular events were significantly reduced with intensive therapy, however the difference in macroalbuminuria is what drives this difference. Indeed, 1.2% of the overall risk difference of 1.9% is contributed by the reduction in macroalbuminuria.[17]

There are a variety of methods that we can use to describe results, and we've included the most important ones in Table 4.14; we'll illustrate them with the help of a randomized trial of statins in patients at risk for stroke. As you can see from the actual trial results in Table 4.4, at a mean of 5 years follow-up, stroke occurred among 5.7% of patients randomized to the control group (we'll call this the "control event rate", CER) and in 4.3% of the patients assigned to receive statin therapy (we'll call this the "experimental event rate", EER). This difference was statistically significant, but how can it be expressed in a clinically useful way? Most often we see this effect reported in clinical journals and the lay press as the relative risk reduction (RRR) calculated as (|CER – EER|/CER). In this example, the RRR is (5.7% – 4.3%)/5.7%, i.e., 25%, and we can say that statin therapy decreased the risk of stroke by 25% relative to those who received placebo.

Table 4.3 Intensive vs standard glucose control to prevent vascular events in type 2 diabetes

Outcomes at median (5 year)	Intensive control (%)	Standard of control (%)	RRR	(95% CI)	NNT	(CI)
Macro- or microvascular event	18	20	9%	2 to 16	56%	31 to 280
Macrovascular event[a]	10	11	6%	−6 to 15	Not significant	
Microvascular event[b]	9.4	11	13%	3 to 22	69%	42 to 324
New or worsening nephropathy[c]	4.1	5.2	21%	7 to 33	94%	58 to 282
Macroalbuminuria	2.9	4.1	30%	15 to 42	83%	58 to 166
New-onset microalbuminuria	24	26	8%	2 to 13	50%	30 to 226
Severe hypoglycemia	2.7	1.5	85%[d]	42 to 137	79%[e]	49 to 161

Abbreviations defined in Glossary. RRR, RRI, NNT, NNH, and CI calculated from data in article.
[a]Non-fatal myocardial infarction (intensive vs standard, 2.7% vs 2.8%), non-fatal stroke (3.8% vs 3.8%), or death from cardiovascular causes (4.5% vs 5.2%).
[b]New or worsening nephropathy or retinopathy (6.0% vs 6.3%).
[c]Macroalbuminuria, doubling of serum creatinine (1.2% vs 1.1%), and renal-replacement therapy or death from renal causes (0.4% vs 0.6%).
[d]RRI.
[e]NNH.
The ADVANCE Collaborative Group. Intensive blood glucose control and vascular outcomes in patients with type 2 diabetes. N Engl J Med 2008; 358: 2560–2572. ACP Journal Club 2008 Sept 16; 149: JC3–6.[16]

4

In a similar way, we can describe the situation in which the experimental treatment increases the risk of a good event as the "relative benefit increase" (RBI; also calculated as |CER – EER|/CER). For example, our study on antipsychotics refers to a recent trial by Schneider and colleagues of atypical antipsychotic drugs in patients with Alzheimer disease.[2] In this randomized trial, 421 patients with the disease and psychosis, aggression or agitation were randomly assigned (with allocation concealment) to receive one of three atypical antipsychotics or placebo. The main outcomes included the number of patients with minimal improvement on the Clinical Global Impression of Change (CGIC) scale at 12 weeks. Analysis was by intention to treat. A total of 29% of patients who were assigned risperidone showed improvement on the CGIC compared with 21% of those allocated to

Table 4.4 Measures of effect size

	Event rate = Stroke (mean follow-up 5 years)		Relative risk reduction (RRR)	Absolute risk reduction (ARR)	Number needed to treat (NNT)
	Control event rate (CER)	Experimental event rate (EER)	|CER – EER|/CER	|CER-EER|	1/ARR
MRC trial	5.7%	4.3%	|5.7 – 4.3%|/5.7% = 25%	|5.7 – 4.3%| = 0.014 or 1.4%	1/1.4% = 72
Hypothetical, trivial case	0.000057%	0.000043%	|0.000057 – 0.000043%| /0.000057% = 25%	|0.000057 – 0.000043%| = 0.000014%	1/0.000014% = 7142857

the placebo group. The relative benefit increase with risperidone is (21% – 29%)/21% or 38%.

If the treatment increases the probability of a bad event, we can use the same formulae to generate the "relative risk increase" (RRI). In the first study of antipsychotics that we found by Ballard and colleagues,[1] mortality at 12 months was not significantly different between the two groups but at 24 months, it was 54% in the group allocated to receive antipsychotic drugs compared with 38% in the placebo group. The relative risk increase was 30%.

One of the disadvantages of the RRR, which makes it unhelpful for our purposes, is revealed in the hypothetical data outlined in the bottom row of Table 4.4. The RRR doesn't reflect the risk of the event without therapy (the CER, or baseline risk) and therefore cannot discriminate huge treatment effects from small ones. For example, if the stroke risk was trivial (0.000057%) in the control group and similarly trivial (0.000043%) in the experimental group, the RRR remains 25%.

One measure that overcomes this lack of discrimination between small and large treatment effects looks at the absolute arithmetic difference between the rates in the two groups. This is called the absolute risk reduction (ARR) (or the risk difference) and it preserves the baseline risk. In the statin trial, the ARR is 5.7% – 4.3% = 1.4%. In our hypothetical case, where the baseline risk is trivial, the ARR is trivial too, at 0.000014%. Thus, the ARR is a more meaningful measure of treatment effects than the RRR. When the experimental treatment increases the probability of a good event, we can generate the absolute benefit increase (ABI), which is also calculated by finding the absolute arithmetic difference in event rates. Similarly, when the experimental treatment increases the probability of a bad event, we can calculate the absolute risk increase (ARI).

The inverse of the ARR (1/ARR) is a whole number and has the useful property of telling us the number of patients that we need to treat (NNT) with the experimental therapy for the duration of the trial in order to prevent one additional bad outcome. In our statin example, the NNT is 1/1.4% = 72, which means we would need to treat 72 people with a statin (rather than placebo) for 5 years to prevent one additional person from suffering a stroke. In our hypothetical example in the bottom row of Table 4.4, the clinical usefulness of the NNT is underscored, for this tiny treatment effect means that we would have to treat over 7 million patients for 5 years to prevent one additional bad event!

The study by Ballard and colleagues[1] doesn't report impact on behavior so we will use the study by Schneider and colleagues[2] to inform this aspect. In this latter study, risperidone therapy led to a relative benefit increase of 30%. We can calculate the NNT using the 29% who obtained benefit in the risperidone group compared with 21% in the placebo group. The risk difference is 8% and this translates to a number needed to treat of 13. We'd need to treat 13 people with risperidone for 12 weeks to see a minimal improvement in the CGIC in one person.

What's a good NNT? We can get an idea by comparing with NNTs for other interventions and durations of therapy, tempered by our own clinical experience and expertise. The smaller the NNT is, the more impressive the result. However, we should also consider the seriousness of the outcome that we are trying to prevent. We've provided some examples of NNTs in Table 4.5. For example, we'd only need to treat 12 people with acute ischemic stroke with alteplase within 4 hours to decrease disability at 1 year. In contrast, we'd have to treat over 100 people with hypertension for 5.5 years to prevent one death, stroke or MI. If you want to see more NNTs, visit our website (www.cebm.utoronto.ca) or take a look at the CD that accompanies this book – you can download some NNT tables to your PDA and nominate an NNT for inclusion on the website.

We can describe the adverse effects of therapy in an analogous fashion, as the number needed to harm one more patient (NNH) from the therapy. The NNH is calculated as 1/ARI. In the statin study, 0.03% of the control group experienced rhabdomyolysis compared with 0.05% of patients who experienced this in the group that received a statin. This absolute risk increase of $|0.03\% - 0.05\%| = 0.02\%$ generates an NNH over 5 years, of 5000. This means that we'd need to treat 5000 patients with a statin for 5 years to cause one additional patient to have rhabdomyolysis. Thus, the NNT and NNH provide us with a nice measure of the effort we and our patients have to expend to prevent or cause one more bad outcome, and their attractiveness as an effort:yield ratio (or "poor clinicians' cost-effectiveness analysis") is easily recognized.

In our study of antipsychotics by Ballard and colleagues,[1] mortality was not significantly different at 12 months. At 24 months, the number needed to harm was found to be 8 – note this number is slightly different than if we calculated it directly from the RRI because it was adjusted for differences between the groups.

Table 4.5 Some useful NNTs[a]

Target disorder	Intervention	Events being prevented	Event rate		Follow-up time	Number needed to treat	Number needed to harm
			Control event rate	Experimental event rate (EER)			
Diastolic blood pressure 115–129 mmHg[b]	Antihypertensive drugs	Death, stroke or MI	13%	1.4%	1.5 years	3	
Diastolic blood pressure 90–109 mmHg[c]	Antihypertensive drugs	Death, stroke or MI	5.5%	4.7%	5.5 years	128	
Symptomatic high-grade carotid stenosis[d]	Carotid endarterectomy (compared with medical therapy)	Death or major stroke	18%	8%	2 years	10	
Acute ischemic stroke[e]	Thrombolysis with alteplase within 3–4.5 hours	Modified Rankin Score 0 to 1	45%	52%	1 year	12	
Acute ischemic stroke[e]	Thrombolysis with alteplase within 3–4.5 hours	Intracranial hemorrhage	18%	27%			11
Type 2 diabetes and microalbuminuria[f]	Multicomponent intervention	All cause mortality	50%	30%	6 months	6	
Type 2 diabetes not treated with insulin[g]	Self-testing	Hypoglycemic episodes	10%	22%			9

[a]Please see: www.cebm.utoronto.ca for additional NNTs
[b]JAMA 1967; 202: 116–122.
[b]BMJ 1995; 291: 97–104.
[c]NEJM 1991; 325: 445–453.
[d]NEJM 2008; 359: 1317–1329.
[e]NEJM 2008; 358: 580–591.
[f]BMJ 2007; 33: 132.

4

To understand NNTs, we need to consider some additional features. First, they always have a dimension of follow-up time associated with them. Quick reference to Table 4.5 reminds us that the NNT of 10 to prevent one more major stroke or death by performing endarterectomy on patients with symptomatic high-grade carotid stenosis refers to outcomes over a 2-year period (in this case, from an operation that is over in minutes). One consequence of this time dimension is that if we want to compare NNTs and NNHs for different follow-up times, we have to make an assumption about them and a "time adjustment" to at least one of them. Say that we wanted to compare the NNTs to prevent one additional stroke, MI or death with drugs among patients with mild vs severe hypertension. Another quick look at Table 4.5 gives us an NNT at 1.5 years of just three for severe hypertensives (who already have a lot of target organ damage) and an NNT at 5.5 years of 128 for milder hypertensives (most of whom are free of target organ damage). To compare their NNTs we need to adjust at least one of them so that they relate to the same follow-up time. The assumption that we make here is that the RRR from antihypertensive therapy is constant over time (i.e., we assume that antihypertensive therapy exerts the same relative benefit in year 1 as it does over the next 4 years). If we are comfortable with that assumption (it appears safe for hypertension), we can then proceed to make the time adjustment.

Let's adjust the NNT for the mild hypertensives (128 over the "observed" 5.5 years) to an NNT corresponding to a "hypothetical" 1.5 years. This is done by multiplying the NNT for the "observed" follow-up time by a fraction with the "observed" time in the numerator and the "hypothetical" time in the denominator. In this case, adjusting the NNT of 128 for mild hypertensives to its hypothetical value for 1.5 years becomes:

$$NNThypothetical = NNTobserved \times (observed\ time\ /\ hypothetical\ time)$$
$$NNT1.5 = 128 \times (5.5\ /\ 1.5) = 470$$

(By convention, we round any decimal NNT upwards to the next whole number.)

Now we can appreciate the vast difference in the yield of clinical efforts to treat mild vs severe hypertensives: we need to treat 470 of the former, but only three of the latter for 1.5 years in order to prevent one additional bad outcome. The explanation lies in the huge difference in CERs (far higher in severe hypertensives followed just 1.5 years than in mild hypertensives followed 5.5 years).

In our antipsychotics example, the study by Schneider and colleagues[2] (which provides our NNT) followed patients to 12 weeks, whereas the study by Ballard (which provides our NNH) followed patients to 24 months. Our adjusted NNT for 24 months = $13 \times (3/24) = 2$.

Second, returning to Table 4.4 and our statin example, we calculated an NNT of 72, but patients can have a different baseline risk of the outcome (depending on the presence of co-morbid illnesses, etc.) and therefore they may be of higher or lower risk of the event than the "average" patient in the study. The NNT can be adjusted for our patient's individual baseline risk of the outcome and this will be discussed later.

2. How precise is this estimate of the treatment effect?

The third thing we need to remember about the NNT is that, like any other clinical measure, NNTs are estimates of the truth and we should specify the limits within which we can confidently state that the true NNT lies (if we want to specify the limits within which the true NNT lies 95% of the time, it's called specifying the 95% "confidence interval"). The confidence interval (CI) provides the range of values that are likely to include the true risk and quantifies the uncertainty in measurement. For example, the PROGRESS trial reported that blood pressure lowering after stroke or TIA reduced the absolute rates of ischemic stroke from 10% to 8% (relative risk reduction (RRR), 24%; 95% confidence interval (CI), 10 to 35). So we have 95% confidence that the true RRR value lies between 10% and 35%, with 24% being the most likely value. The absolute risk reduction is 2% (from 10% to 8%), for which we can also calculate a 95% CI from 1% to 3.5% (using the 10% control group rate and the 95% CI for the RRR). Finally, we can calculate the CI for the NNT by simply taking the inverse of the absolute risk's confidence intervals: 1/0.01 and 1/0.035. Thus, the 95% CI for the NNT is 100 to 29. The smaller the number of patients in the study that generated the NNT, the wider its CI, but even when the CI is wide, it can provide us with some guidance and we should look at the limits of the CI. In the PROGRESS trial example, the trial shows a positive effect but we need look at the upper limit of the CI for the NNT. Is the value of 100 clinically important? If we decide that it isn't, the study results are unhelpful, even although it is statistically significant (that is $p < 0.05$). Similarly, if the study results are negative, we can look at the limits of the CI to see if a potentially important positive benefit has been excluded. A result that isn't statistically significant (that is $p > 0.05$) can still be helpful to us! Incidentally, confidence intervals and p values are closely related (see below).

Confidence intervals and significance tests are closely related. Generally a "significant" *p* value of *p* < 0.05 will correspond to a 95% CI, which excludes the value indicating no difference. The "no difference" value is 0 for a difference of measures (such as absolute risk difference, difference in blood pressure, etc.) and is 1 for a ratio (such as the relative risk, odds ratio, or hazard ratio).

For example, an absolute risk difference of 5% (95% CI −5% to +15%) is not statistically significant because the 95% CI includes 0, whereas a risk difference of 5% (95% CI 2–8%) would be statistically significant because it does not include 0. Similarly, a relative risk of 0.80 (95% CI 0.50–1.1) would not be statistically significant because it includes 1, whereas a relative risk of 0.80 (95% CI 0.70– 0.90) would be statistically significant because it does not include 1 (the "no effect" value for ratio measures).

Most statisticians now agree that estimation, including confidence intervals, are preferable for summarizing the results of a study, but CIs and *p* values are complementary and many papers present both.

(For details on calculating CIs, see the accompanying CD and www. cebm.utoronto.ca).

Practicing EBM in real-time: calculating the measures of treatment effect – a shortcut

Rather than memorizing the formula described above, we could instead use an EBM calculator whenever we need to calculate the measure of the treatment effect (i.e., if the results of the study aren't presented in the article using these measures). This tool saves us time and decreases the risk of a mathematical error. From our website and from the accompanying CD you can download an EBM calculator that we've developed (www.cebm.utoronto.ca/practice/ca/statscal/) and this calculator can also be downloaded to your PDA.

Let's try to repeat the calculations that we completed in Table 4.4. In the dropdown box on the calculator, click on the RCT option. We can enter the data from the table and at a click of a button we can obtain the measures of effect and their confidence intervals (see Figure 4.2).

When retrieving evidence, we also completed a search of *ACP Journal Club* and identified an entry for the study by Ballard and colleagues.[18] We know that this article has passed some quality filters since it appears in this journal (Ch. 2) and it has been rated on clinical relevance and newsworthiness by clinicians. Contrast this more informative abstract with that from the original article. We can quickly see that it was a randomized, placebo-controlled study in which patients, and caregivers, clinicians, those who administered the medication, and outcomes assessors were blinded. The investigators used an intention to

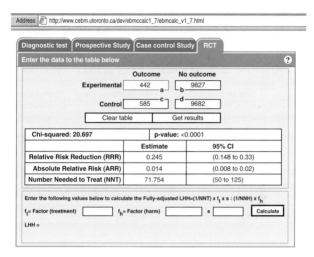

Figure 4.2 Practicing EBM in real-time: Using pre-appraised evidence.

4

treat analysis and 100% follow-up was achieved. Of note, a declarative title and the clinical question that the trial addressed (using the PICO format) are included. Using the *ACP Journal Club* abstract we can appraise the trial's validity and importance in less than a minute and quickly move to decide if we can apply the evidence to our patient. Moreover, there is a commentary by an expert clinician who provides a clinical bottom line and places the evidence from this article in context with other evidence.

We can also find this article in a search of *Evidence Updates*. Indeed, we had already seen this article in a weekly e-mail we receive and we had saved it to our own, searchable database within *Evidence Updates*. We were able to retrieve the citation, adapted in Figure 4.3. The citation includes comments from clinicians from primary care, geriatric medicine and neurology. Comments on study quality and clinical context which appear may help us in our interpretation and use of the evidence.

Are the valid, important results of this individual study applicable to our patient?

Now that we have decided that the evidence we have found is both valid and important, we need to consider if we can apply it to our own patient.

Quick search

Search term(s):

dementia and antipsychotics

☐ Use my clinical discipline(s) ⦿ Order by most recent ○ Order by best match

Ballard C, Hanney ML, Theodoulou M, et al. **The dementia antipsychotic withdrawal trial (DART-AD): long term follow-up of a randomised placebo-controlled trial.** Lancet Neurol. 2009 Feb;8(2): 151-7. Epub 2009 Jan 8. (Original) PMID: 19138567

Read Abstract   Read Comments

DISCIPLINE	RELEVANCE TO PRACTICE	IS THIS NEWS?
General Internal Medicine–Primary Care (US)	■■■■■■☐	■■■■■■☐
General Practice (GP) Family Practice (FP)	■■■■■■☐	■■■■■■☐
Geriatrics	■■■■■■■	■■■■■■☐
Neurology	■■■■■■☐	■■■■■■☐

Abstract

BACKGROUND: Data from 12-week placebo-controlled trials have led to mounting concerns about increased mortality in patients with Alzheimer's disease (AD) who are prescribed antipsychotics; however, there are no mortality data from long-term placebo-controlled trials. We aimed to assess whether continued treatment with antipsychotics in people with AD is associated with an increased risk of mortality.

METHODS: Between October, 2001, and December, 2004, patients with AD who resided in care facilities in the UK were enrolled into a randomised, placebo-controlled, parallel, two-group treatment discontinuances trial. Participants were randomly assigned to continue with their antipsychotic treatment (thioridazine, chlorpromazine, haloperidol, trifluoperazine, or risperidone) for 12 months or to switch their medication to an oral placebo. The primary outcome was mortality at 12 months. An additional follow-up telephone assessment was done to establish whether each participant was still alive 24 months after the enrollment of the last participant (range 24-25 months). Causes of death were obtained from death certificates. Analysis

Figure 4.3 *Evidence Updates* screenshot. Comments on study quality and clinical context which appear may help us in our interpretation and use of the evidence.

To apply evidence, we need to integrate the evidence with our clinical experience and expertise, and with our patient's values and preferences. The guides for doing this are in Table 4.6.

1. Is our patient so different from those in the study that its results cannot apply?

We need to use our clinical expertise to decide if our patient is so different from those in the study that its results don't apply. One approach

CARDS

Table 4.6 Is this valid and important evidence (from an individual randomized trial) applicable to our patient?

1. Is our patient so different from those in the study that its results cannot apply?
2. Is the treatment feasible in our setting?
3. What are our patient's potential benefits and harms from the therapy?
4. What are our patient's values and expectations for both the outcome we are trying to prevent and the treatment we are offering?

would be to demand that our patient fit all the inclusion criteria for the study and reject it if our patient doesn't fit each one. This isn't a very sensible approach because most differences between our patients and those in trials tend to be quantitative (they have different ages or different degrees of risk of the outcome event or of responsiveness to the therapy) rather than qualitative (total absence of responsiveness to treatment or risk of event). We'd suggest that a more appropriate approach is to consider whether our patient's sociodemographic features or pathobiology are so different from those in the study that its results are useless to us and our patient; only then should we discard its results and resume our search for relevant evidence. There are only a few occasions when this might be the case: different pharmacogenetics, absent immune responses, co-morbid conditions that prohibit the treatment, and the like. As a consequence of this clinical (as opposed to actuarial) approach, it's rare that we have to toss away a study for this reason. One difference we do need to consider is whether our patient is likely to accept our advice and comply with the demands of the therapeutic regimen, and we'll address that at the end of this section.

Sometimes treatments appear to produce qualitative differences in the responses of subgroups of patients so that they appear to benefit some subgroups but not others. Such qualitative differences in responses are extremely rare. For example, some early trials of aspirin for transient ischemic attacks showed large benefits for men but none for women; subsequent trials and systematic reviews showed that this was a chance finding and that aspirin is efficacious in women. If you think that the treatment you're examining may work in a qualitatively different way among different subgroups of patients, you should refer to the guides in Table 4.7. To summarize them, unless the difference in response makes biological sense, was hypothesized before the trial, and has been confirmed in a second, independent trial, we'd suggest that you accept the treatment's overall efficacy as the best starting point for estimating its efficacy in your individual patient.

In the study of antipsychotic drugs by Schneider and colleagues,[2] it is suggested that patients who have more severe behavioral disturbances might achieve more benefit from these agents. This has not been confirmed in a meta-analysis of trials.

Table 4.7 Guides for whether to believe apparent qualitative differences in the efficacy of therapy in some subgroups of patients

A qualitative difference in treatment efficacy among subgroups is likely only when ALL the following questions can be answered "yes":
1. Does it really make biological and clinical sense?
2. Is the qualitative difference both clinically (beneficial for some but useless or harmful for others) and statistically significant?
3. Was it hypothesized before the study began (rather than the product of dredging the data)?
4. Was it one of just a few subgroup analyses carried out in the study?
5. Is this subgroup difference suggested by comparisons within rather than between studies?
6. Has the result been confirmed in other independent studies?

2. Is the treatment feasible in our setting?

Next we need to consider if the treatment is feasible in our practice setting. Can our patient, or healthcare system pay for the treatment, its administration and the required monitoring? Is the treatment available in our setting? Antipsychotic therapies are variable in cost – with some of the newer agents being quite expensive. However, in a long-term care facility, these costs would usually be covered.

3. What are our patient's potential benefits and harms from the therapy?

After we have decided that the study is applicable to our patients and that the treatment is feasible, we need to estimate our patient's unique benefits and risks of therapy. There are two general approaches to doing this. The first and longer approach begins by coming up with the best possible estimate of what would happen to our patient if he were not treated, his individual CER or "patient's expected event rate" (PEER). To this estimate we can apply the overall RRR (for the events we hope to prevent with therapy) and RRI (for the adverse effects of therapy) and generate the corresponding NNT and NNH for our specific patient. The second, much quicker approach skips this PEER step and works entirely from the NNT and NNH in the study. Note that with both approaches, we assume that the relative benefits and risks of therapy are the same for patients with high and low PEERs. Because the second method is so much quicker, you might want to skip to that method, but if you want to learn the long way first, read on.

The long way, via PEER

There are four ways to estimate our patient's PEER. First, we can simply assign our patient the overall CER from the study; this is easy, but sensible only if our patient is the "average" study patient. Second, if the study has a subgroup of patients with characteristics similar to our own patient, we can assign to him the CER for that subgroup. (Indeed, in the unlikely event that we could say "yes" to all of the questions posed in Table 4.13, we could even apply the ARR for that subgroup to generate an NNT for our patient.) Third, if the study report includes a valid clinical prediction guide, we could use it to assign a PEER to our patient. Fourth, we could look for another paper that described the prognosis of untreated patients like ours and use its results to assign our patient a PEER. All four methods we've described generate a PEER for our patient – what we would expect to happen to them if they received the "control" or comparison intervention in the study we're using. To convert this into an NNT or NNH for patients just like ours, we have to apply the corresponding RRR and RRI to them, using the formula:

$$NNT = 1 / (PEER \times RRR) \text{ or}$$
$$NNH = 1 / (PEER \times RRI)$$

4

For example, suppose that we find a paper that suggests that our patient with Alzheimer disease has a risk of death of 30% over 2 years given his cardiac history and Alzheimer disease (so his PEER is 30%). The trial by Ballard and colleagues[2] generated an overall adjusted RRI of 36% at 24–54 months, so the NNH for patients like ours is $1/(30\% \times 36\%) = 9$. Similarly, we could adjust the NNT if we think our patient's risk of benefit from antipsychotics is different from that in the study using:

$$NNT = 1 / (PEER \times RBI).$$

As you can see, these calculations can be cumbersome to do without a calculator, and fortunately Dr G Chatellier and his colleagues published the convenient nomogram shown in Figure 4.4 to help us. Alternatively, we could use the EBM calculator from our website (www. cebm.utoronto.ca).

The short way, sticking with NNT/NNH

This is a faster and easier method of estimating an NNT or NNH for our patient and is the one we usually use at the bedside or in the clinic. In this approach, the estimate we make for our patient's risk of the outcome

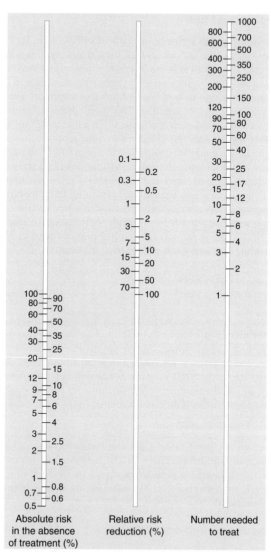

Figure 4.4 Nomogram for determining NNTs. (From Chatellier G, Zapletal E, Lemaitre D, et al. The number needed to treat: a clinically useful nomogram in its proper context. BMJ 1996; 312: 426–9)

event (if the patient were to receive just the "control" therapy) is specified relative to that of the average control patient, and expressed as a "decimal fraction" we call f_t. For example, if we think that our patient (if left untreated) has twice the risk of the outcome as control patients in the trial, $f_t = 2$; alternatively, if we think our patient is at only half their risk, then $f_t = 0.5$. We can use our past clinical experience and expertise in coming up with a value for f_t or we can use any of the information sources described in the previous section. Remembering our assumption that the treatment produces a constant relative risk reduction across the range of susceptibilities, the NNT for patients just like ours is simply the reported NNT divided by f_t. In our statin example, we calculated an NNT of 72, so we'd need to treat 72 patients like those in the trial with a statin for a mean of 5 years to prevent one more of them from experiencing a stroke. If, however, we judge that our patient is at three times the risk of stroke without treatment as the patients in the control group, $f_t = 3$ and $NNT/f_t = 72/3 = 24$. This means that we would only need to treat 24 higher-risk patients like ours for 5 years to prevent an additional stroke.

Again, we need to consider our patient's risk of adverse events from the therapy and to do this, we can use any of the same methods that we used to individualize our patient's NNT. Using the simplest one, we may decide that our patient is at three times the risk of adverse events as patients in the control group of the study ($f_h = 3$), or we may decide that our patient is at one-third the risk ($f_h = 0.33$). Assuming the RRI of harm is constant over the spectrum of susceptibilities, we can adjust the study NNH of 5000 with f_h (just as we did for the NNT), and generate NNH values of 1667 and 15 152 corresponding to f_h values of 3 and 0.33, respectively.

> Returning to our antipsychotic study, we may believe that our patient's risk of death was greater than those in the control group – indeed given his history of CAD, we imagine it is three times that of the control group, f_h is therefore 3 and the NNH becomes 9/3 or 3. We'd only need to treat three people like our patient to cause one additional death.

4. What are our patient's values and expectations for both the outcome we are trying to prevent and the treatment we are offering?

Thus far we've individualized the benefits and risks of therapy for our patient but we've ignored his values and preferences. How can we incorporate these into a treatment recommendation? More importantly, how can we convert these into a form that permits our patient to make his own treatment decision? There are several models available for providing shared decision-making support including elaborate ("Rolls Royce") ways of doing this, such as a formal clinical decision analysis (CDA) which incorporates the patient's likelihood of the outcome events with their own values for each health state. However, performing a clinical decision analysis for each patient would be too time-consuming for the busy clinician and patient and this approach therefore usually relies on finding an existing decision analysis. To be able to use the existing decision analysis (we'll discuss this in a later section), either our patient's values (and risks) must approximate those in the analysis, or the decision analysis must provide information about the impact of variation in patient values (and risks) on the results of the decision analysis. And, even expert clinical decision analysts find them prohibitively slow to use in the real world. Clinicians can also use validated decision aids that present descriptive and probabilistic information about the target disorder, management options and outcome events to facilitate shared decision-making. But, to date, well-validated decision aids can be tough to find. If you're interested in finding some, take a look at Dr O'Connor's (Ottawa Hospital Research Institute, OHRI) website at: http://decisionaid.ohri.ca/decaids.html.

Is there some quick way of incorporating patient values (say, a "Ka" version) that doesn't do too much violence to the truth?

In an attempt to meet the needs of comprehensibility, applicability and ease of use on busy clinical services, we proposed a patient-centered measure of the likelihood of being helped and harmed by an intervention based on the NNT for target events produced by the intervention (as an expression of the likelihood of being helped), the NNH for the adverse effects of therapy (to express the likelihood of being harmed) and their ratio. This result, when adjusted by an individual patient-centered conviction about the relative severities of these two events, provides an understandable, quality-adjusted, rapidly calculated measure of the likelihood of being helped and harmed (LHH) by a particular therapy. It goes like this:

Returning to our patient with dementia 3, we found that the NNT, adjusted to 24 months, was 2. We could use this to tell our patient's daughter that he has a 1 in 2 chance of being helped by an antipsychotic drug and improved behavior. Similarly, looking at his risk of harm, we could tell him and his daughter that he has a 1 in 9 chance of experiencing harm (death) with this therapy. Our first approximation of his likelihood of being helped vs harmed then becomes:

$$LHH = (1 / NNT) : (1 / NNH)^{\S}$$
$$= (1 / 2) : (1 / 9)$$
$$= 5$$

We could then tell our patient that antipsychotic therapy is five times more likely to help him than to harm him. But, again this ignores his unique risks of benefit and harm from therapy. We might think that his baseline risk of death is higher than that of patients in the control group given his age and co-morbidities (and as in the previous section, we have several options for determining his PEER but for now, we'll stick with the f_t method). We could estimate f_h from our clinical experience and might decide that his risk of death is three times higher ($f_h = 3$) than that of the control patients and similarly we might think his risk of improved behavior was lower than that of the control group (let's say $f_t = 0.33$). His LHH now becomes:

$$LHH = (1 / NNT) \times f_t : (1 / NNH) \times f_h$$
$$= (1 / 2) \times 3 : (1 / 9) \times 0.33$$
$$= 2$$

This now means that our patient is two times more likely to be harmed than helped by the therapy – note that the decision has reversed. *(Note we multiply, rather than divide, by f_t in this case because we are adjusting 1/NNT).*

We now tell our patient and his daughter that based on his unique risks of benefit and harm, he's two times more likely to be harmed than helped by the therapy.

But, this doesn't incorporate our patient's unique values and preferences, the consideration of which leads us to the most critical step in calculating the LHH – eliciting our patient's preferences. We ask our patient (or in our example, his daughter who is his substitute decision-maker) to make value judgments about the relative severity of the bad outcome we hope to prevent with therapy and the adverse event we might cause with it. We begin this in the time-honored way of describing both of them, repeating these descriptions as needed after our patient has had the chance to think about them, and discuss them with family members, etc. When the treatment option is a common one (on our service, whether to take long-term warfarin for non-valvular atrial fibrillation),

---

§Note that we could also say LHH = ARR : ARI

we might conclude our discussion by leaving our patient with a written description of the outcomes of foregoing or accepting the treatment.

Following the review of these descriptions of the target event we hope to prevent and the adverse effects we might cause, we work with the patient to help him express how severe he considers one of them relative to the other – is death 20 times as severe as the agitation? Five times as severe? This can be accomplished in a quick and simple way by asking our patient (or his decision-maker) to tell us which is worse, and by how much. If the patient has difficulty making this comparison in a direct fashion, we present him/her with a rating scale (Figure 4.5), the ends of which are anchored at 0 (= death or stroke or ??**) and 1 (= full health). Next, we ask our patient to place a mark where he would consider the value of the target event we hope to prevent with treatment (our patient's daughter assigned death a value of 0.025). Similarly, we ask her to place a second mark to correspond with the value for the behavior (agitation, aggression) we are trying to prevent (our patient's daughter assigned the adverse events a value of 0.95, only a minor "disutility"). Comparing these two ratings, we can say that our patient believes that death is 38 (0.95/0.025) times worse than the agitation we are trying to avoid (we call this relative value the severity or "s" factor). We then ask her whether this comparison makes sense, and usually repeat this process on a second occasion to see whether this relative severity is stable.

Integrating this with our risk-adjusted LHH, the LHH becomes:

$$[(1 / NNT) \times f_t] : [(1 / NNH) \times f_h \times s]$$
$$= [(1 / 2) \times 3 \times 38] : [(1 / 9) \times 0.33 \times 19]$$
$$= 38$$

Thus, in the final analysis, our patient is 38 times as likely to be harmed vs helped by antipsychotic therapy.

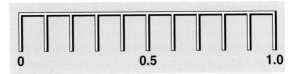

Figure 4.5 Rating scale for assessing values.

**Yes, our patients sometimes identify fates worse than death, in which case we extend the line below 0.

(Instead of using the "s" factor, we could incorporate our patient's utilities directly into the LHH:

$$LHH = (1 / NNT) \times f_t \times (1 - U_{event}) : (1 / NNH) \times (1 - U_{toxicity}) \times f_h$$
$$= (1 / 2) \times (1 - 0.05) \times 3 : (1 / 9) \times (1 - 0.975) \times 0.33)$$
$$= 38$$

(Note that 1 – Utility provides the "disutility" associated with the outcome).

If we are unsure of our patient's "f" for benefit or harm, or if our patient is uncertain about his "severity" factor, we can do a sensitivity analysis by inserting other clinically sensible values for "f" and "s" and see how they affect the size and direction of the LHH.

The foregoing discussion demonstrates the "Ka" model of the LHH, but it is a far cry from the "Rolls Royce" of clinical decision analysis. We could add a few features to the basic LHH, making it into a Jaguar that can compare two active treatments (instead of just a placebo vs experimental treatment, as in our example). If there were several serious adverse events that could result from the treatment(s), we could add each of them to generate the fully adjusted LHH. Finally, as we will describe later in this chapter, we can also discount future events as in a CDA.

4

We've found that the LHH can be used in the busy clinical setting (median time to complete of 6.5 min), is intelligible to both clinicians and patients, and is unambiguously patient-centered. A version of the LHH is available on the accompanying CD. Take a crack at downloading it to your PDA and let us know what you think. As other approaches in this rapidly developing field are validated in clinical settings, they will appear on our website and in future editions of this book.

Now that we've completed a critical appraisal of the paper that we retrieved, we may want to keep a permanent record of this. We find that CATs are most useful as teaching tools. CATbanks are great practice tools if we can find sites that describe and use rigorous methodology for the creation, peer review and updating of CATs. However, these tasks require tremendous resources and few CATbanks that we've found meet these needs.

Further reading about individual randomized trials

Guyatt G, Rennie D, Meade M, Cook DJ, eds. *Users' guides to the medical literature. A manual for evidence-based clinical practice.* Chicago: AMA Press; 2008.

Haynes RB, Sackett DL, Guyatt GH, et al. *Clinical epidemiology: How to do clinical practice research*. Philadelphia: Lippincott Williams & Wilkins; 2006.

Straus SE. Individualizing treatment decisions: the likelihood of being helped versus harmed. *Eval Health Prof*. 2002;25(2):210–224.

Reports of systematic reviews

It might appear that this section is out of order because the first target of any search about therapy should be a systematic review since it is the most powerful and useful evidence available. However, because the critical appraisal of a systematic review requires the skill to appraise the individual trials that comprise it, we've switched the order in this book.

A systematic review (SR) is a summary of the clinical literature that uses explicit methods to systematically search, critically appraise, and synthesize the world literature on a specific issue. Its goal is to minimize both bias (usually by not only restricting itself to randomized trials, but also seeking published and unpublished reports in every language) and random error (by amassing very large numbers of individuals). SRs may, but need not, include some statistical method for combining the results of individual studies (and we'll call this subset "meta-analyses"). In contrast, traditional literature reviews usually don't include an exhaustive literature search or synthesis of studies. The guides that we consider when appraising a SR follow. Not surprisingly, many of them (especially around importance and applicability) are the same as those for individual reports, but those for validity are different. We'll start with assessing validity using the guides in Table 4.8; the guides for considering the importance of the results are outlined in Table 4.9.

We see a patient in the preoperative assessment clinic. He is a 72-year-old man with a history of hypertension and stroke who is on a diuretic, a statin and ASA. He is awaiting an elective hip replacement. The resident in our clinic wonders whether this patient should receive a beta-blocker medication in the perioperative period. Together we formulate the question: in a patient undergoing elective hip replacement, does treatment with a beta-blocker decrease his risk of death, stroke and cardiac events? We search PubMed Clinical Queries using the terms "beta antagonist" and "surgery" and we retrieve a systematic review by Bangalore and colleagues, published in 2008.[19]

Table 4.8 Is the evidence from this systematic review valid?

1. Is this a systematic review of randomized trials?
2. Does it describe a comprehensive and detailed search for relevant trials?
3. Were the individual studies assessed for validity?

A less frequent point:

4. Were individual patient data (or aggregate data) used in the analysis?

Table 4.9 Is the valid evidence from this systematic review important?

1. Are the results consistent across studies?
2. What is the magnitude of the treatment effect?
3. How precise is the treatment effect?

Are the results of this systematic review valid?

1. Is this a systematic review of randomized trials?

Initially we need to determine whether the systematic review combines randomized or non-randomized trials. SRs, by combining all relevant randomized trials, reduce both bias and random error and thus provide the highest level of evidence currently achievable about the effects of healthcare.[††] In contrast, systematic reviews of non-randomized trials can compound the problems of individually misleading trials and produce a lower quality of evidence. For this reason, if the SR we find includes both randomized and non-randomized trials, we avoid it unless it separates these types of trials in its analyses.

> Our review includes randomized trials investigating the use of beta-blockers in patients undergoing non-cardiac surgery.

[††]This is why the Cochrane Collaboration has been compared with the Human Genome Project, however, we think that the Cochrane Collaboration faces a greater challenge given the infinite number of trials vs the finite number of genes! Mallett and Clarke have suggested at least 10 000 systematic reviews are needed to cover studies relevant to healthcare as identified by the Cochrane Collaboration in 2003. (Mallett S, Clarke M. How many Cochrane reviews are needed to cover existing evidence on the effects of health care interventions? ACP J Club 2003; 139: A11).

2. Does it describe a comprehensive and detailed search for relevant trials?

We need to scrutinize the Methods section to determine whether it describes how the investigators found all the relevant trials. If not, we drop it and continue looking. If they did carry out a search, we seek reassurance that it went beyond standard bibliographic databases, as these have been shown to fail to label correctly up to half of the published trials in their files. A more rigorous SR would include hand-searching journals, conference proceedings, theses, and the databanks of pharmaceutical firms, as well as contacting authors of published articles. Negative trials are less likely to be submitted and selected for publication (which could result in a false-positive conclusion in a SR restricted to published trials) and the other sources regularly turn up less enthusiastic unpublished trials. And if the SR's authors restricted their search to reports in just one language, this, too, could bias the conclusions. It has been observed, for example, that bilingual German investigators were more likely to submit trials with positive results to English language journals and those with negative results to German language journals.[‡‡] More journals are now requiring authors to identify the impact on the results of excluding studies due to language restrictions. And, as with reporting of individual trials, journals are asking for a flow diagram (outlined in the PRISMA statement[20] aimed at enhancing accuracy of reporting of reviews) to illustrate the yield from the search and appraisal process. Figure 4.6 illustrates the flow diagram for the study we found.

> The authors of our review searched PubMed, EMBASE, and the Cochrane Library from 1966 to May 2008. They also searched references of retrieved articles. There is no mention of language restrictions.

3. Were the individual studies assessed for validity?

The methods section of the report should also include a statement describing how the investigators assessed the validity of the individual studies (using criteria like those in Table 4.1). We would feel most confident in the systematic review in which multiple independent reviews of individual studies were carried out and showed good agreement.

[‡‡]This observation applies to allopathic interventions; the situation is reversed for trials assessing complementary medical therapies!

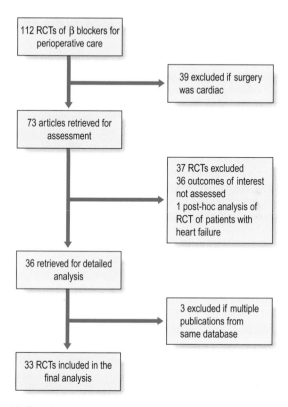

Figure 4.6 Flow diagram for a systematic review. (From Bangalore et al.[19])

At each stage of the review process, we'd like to see that independent assessment was completed, for example, the titles and abstracts of the retrieved articles should be reviewed independently by two investigators to determine if they meet inclusion criteria.

In the review we found, the authors used the quality assessment methods recommended by the Cochrane Collaboration and included consideration of the sequence generation of allocation, allocation concealment, masking of participants, personnel and outcomes assessors, incomplete outcome data, selective outcome reporting, and other sources of bias. Three people independently assessed quality and completed data abstraction.

4. Were individual patient data (or aggregate data) used for the analysis?

A less frequent point to consider is whether the authors used individual patient data (rather than summary tables or published reports) for their analysis. We'd feel more confident about the conclusions of the study, especially as it related to subgroups, if individual patient data were used, because they provide the opportunity to test promising subgroups from one trial in an identical subgroup from other trials (you might want to refer back to Table 4.7). Individual patient data allow more reliable analyses of patients' time to specific clinical events. Individual patient data analysis also allows for more accurate subgroup analysis and ensures appropriateness of follow-up and analysis. Analysis of published, aggregate data can give different answers to an individual patient data meta-analysis because of exclusion of trials, of patients, and differences in length of follow-up, among other factors.

Once we're satisfied with the validity of the SR, we can turn to its results. Table 4.9 outlines the guides that we can use.

Are the valid results of this systematic review important?

1. Are the results consistent across studies?

Were the effects of treatment consistent from study to study? We're more likely to believe the results of a systematic review if the results of every trial included showed a treatment effect that is going in the same direction (what we'd call "qualitatively" similar results). We shouldn't expect them to show exactly the same degree of efficacy (or "quantitatively" identical results), but we should be concerned if some trials confidently conclude a beneficial effect of treatment and others in the same review powerfully exclude any benefit or demonstrate a clear-cut harm. If we look at the all-cause mortality results of the trials with low risk of bias in Figure 4.7 we can first see that five trials are not statistically significant (the CIs overlap with 1, see above), but that two trials are statistically significant (the CIs of MaVS and POISE do not include 1) but in opposite directions! This should make us a little concerned about inconsistency. More generally, we can look at the degree to which the CIs overlap from the various trials. Ideally, we'd like to find that the investigators tested their results to see whether any lack of consistency (or "heterogeneity") was unlikely to be due to the play of chance. And, if they did find statistically significant heterogeneity, did they satisfactorily explain why it was observed (as differences in study patients, in doses of medications, in durations of therapy,

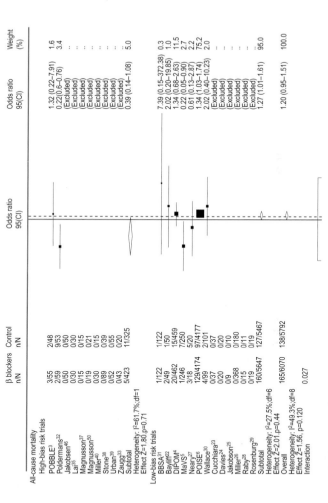

	β blockers n/N	Control n/N	Odds ratio 95(CI)		Odds ratio 95(CI)	Weight (%)
All-cause mortality						
High-bias risk trials						
POBBLE[3]	3/55	2/48			1.32 (0.22–7.91)	1.6
Poldermans[32]	2/59	9/53			0.22(0.6–0.76)	3.4
Jakobsen[46]	0/50	0/50			(Excluded)	:
Lai[35]	0/30	0/30			(Excluded)	:
Magnusson[37]	0/15	0/15			(Excluded)	:
Magnusson[50]	0/19	0/21			(Excluded)	:
Miller[40]	0/30	0/15			(Excluded)	:
Stone[38]	0/89	0/39			(Excluded)	:
Urban[39]	0/52	0/55			(Excluded)	:
Zaugg[33]	0/43	0/20			(Excluded)	:
Subtotal	5/423	11/325			0.39 (0.14–1.08)	5.0
Heterogeneity: I²=61.7%;df=1						
Effect Z=1.80,p=0.71						
Low-bias risk trials						
BBSA[31]	1/122	1/122			7.39 (0.15–372.38)	0.3
Bayliff[22]	2/49	1/50			2.02 (0.20–19.85)	1.0
DIPOM[4]	20/462	15/459			1.34 (0.68–2.63)	11.5
MaVS[5]	1/246	7/250			0.22 (0.05–0.90)	2.7
Neary[27]	3/18	5/20			0.61 (0.13–2.87)	2.2
POISE[6]	129/4174	97/4177			1.34 (1.03–1.74)	75.2
Wallace[30]	4/99	2/101			2.02 (0.40–10.23)	2.0
Cucchiara[23]	0/37	0/37			(Excluded)	:
Davies[24]	0/20	0/20			(Excluded)	:
Jakobson[25]	0/9	0/10			(Excluded)	:
Miller[26]	0/368	0/180			(Excluded)	:
Raby[28]	0/15	0/11			(Excluded)	:
Rosenburg[29]	0/19	0/19			(Excluded)	:
Subtotal	160/5647	127/5467			1.27 (1.01–1.61)	95.0
Heterogeneity: I²=27.5%;df=6						
Effect Z=2.01,p=0.44						
Overall	165/6070	138/5792			1.20 (0.95–1.51)	100.0
Heterogeneity: I²=49.3%;df=8						
Effect Z=1.56, p=0.120						
Interaction	0.027					

Figure 4.7 A Forest Plot.

(Continued)

4

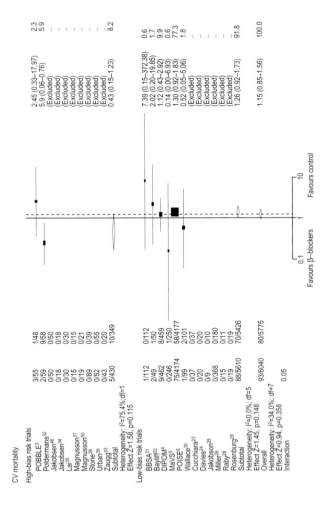

CV mortality

High-bias risk trials

POBBLE[3]	3/55	1/48	2.45 (0.33–17.97)	2.3
Poldermans[32]	2/59	9/58	5.9 (0.06–0.76)	5.9
Jakobsen[46]	0/50	0/50	(Excluded)	
Jakobsen[34]	0/18	0/18	(Excluded)	
Lai[35]	0/30	0/30	(Excluded)	
Magnusson[37]	0/15	0/15	(Excluded)	
Magnusson[50]	0/19	0/21	(Excluded)	
Stone[38]	0/89	0/39	(Excluded)	
Urban[39]	0/52	0/55	(Excluded)	
Zaugg[33]	0/43	0/20	(Excluded)	
Subtotal	5/430	10/349	0.43 (0.15–1.23)	8.2

Heterogeneity: I²=75.4%, df=1
Effect Z=1.58, p=0.115

Low-bias risk trials

BBSA[31]	1/112	0/112	7.39 (0.15–372.38)	0.6
Bayliff[22]	2/49	1/50	2.02 (0.20–19.85)	1.7
DIPOM[4]	9/462	8/459	1.12 (0.43–2.92)	9.9
MaVS[5]	0/246	1/250	0.14 (0.00–6.93)	0.6
POISE[6]	75/4174	58/4177	1.30 (0.92–1.83)	77.3
Wallace[30]	1/99	2/101	0.52 (0.05–5.06)	1.8
Cucchiara[23]	0/37	0/37	(Excluded)	
Davies[24]	0/20	0/20	(Excluded)	
Jakobson[25]	0/9	0/10	(Excluded)	
Miller[26]	0/368	0/180	(Excluded)	
Raby[28]	0/15	0/11	(Excluded)	
Rosenburg[29]	0/19	0/19	(Excluded)	
Subtotal	88/5610	70/5426	1.26 (0.92–1.73)	91.8

Heterogeneity: I²=0.0%, df=5
Effect Z=1.45, p=0.148

| Overall | 93/6040 | 80/5775 | 1.15 (0.85–1.56) | 100.0 |

Heterogeneity: I²=34.0%; df=7
Effect Z=0.94, p=0.358
Interaction 0.05

Favours β–blockers   Favours control

0.1   1   10

Figure 4.7 Cont'd.

outcome measurement, etc.)? If study results are consistent, it is possible for the authors to use statistical methods to summarize the results and this is called meta-analysis. Even if statistical heterogeneity occurs, investigators can complete a meta-analysis; however, it is important for the investigators to explore the impact of this heterogeneity on the meta-analysis.

> In the study we found, heterogeneity was assessed by the I^2 statistic. This refers to the proportion of total variation observed between the trials that is attributable to differences between trials rather than sampling error. The authors regarded an I^2 of 25% as low and 75% or more as high. Clinical heterogeneity was present across trials with differences in patient characteristics, beta-blocker used, and dose, timing and duration of drug use. Sensitivity analyses were completed to determine the impact of heterogeneity on the results. Some 80% of deaths, MIs and strokes came from a single trial which used a relatively high dose of metoprolol. However, the risk of stroke was increased regardless of whether or not this study was included in the meta-analysis.

2. What is the magnitude of the treatment effect?

Just as we examined the results of single therapeutic trials, we need to find a clinically useful expression for the results of systematic reviews, and here we become victims of history and some high-level statistics (the toughest in this book). Although growing numbers of SRs present their results as NNTs, most of them still use odds ratios (ORs) or relative risks (RRs).[§§] Earlier in this chapter, we showed that the RRR doesn't preserve the control event rate (CER) or the patient's expected event rate (PEER), and this disadvantage extends to ORs and RRs. Systematic reviews often present results as a Forest Plot (Figure 4.7) A Forest Plot is a graphical representation of the estimate of treatment effect and its CI. It is particularly helpful in systematic reviews because the authors can include the OR (and CI) for each individual study, as well as the pooled result (which is the result of the meta-analysis). Starting from the left of Figure 4.7, each citation is presented followed by the results from each intervention arm within each study, the OR and the CI. The key things to focus on in these figures (described in detail in Ch. 7) are the line of no difference and the extent of the CI. The line of no difference is drawn for an OR of 1 (the numerator and the denominator are the same thing, the OR is 1, and therefore there

---

[§§]An odds ratio is the odds of an event in a patient in the experimental group relative to that of a patient in the control group. Relative risk is the risk of an event in a patient in the experimental group relative to that of a patient in the control group.

is no difference in the treatment effects). Then we can look to see if the estimate of the OR (for each individual study and for the summary estimate) falls to the left or right of this line and whether the CI for this estimate crosses this line. In Figure 4.7, when the OR and its CI lie to the left of the line of no difference, this means that mortality is decreased with beta-blockers. If the OR and its CI fall to the right of the line of no difference, this means that mortality is increased with beta-blockers and this would favor the control therapy. Fortunately, although ORs and RRs are of very limited use in the clinical setting, they can be converted to NNTs (or NNHs) using the formulae in Table 4.10. Better yet, we've provided the results of some typical conversions in Table 4.11 and Table 4.12. And finally, we can take a shortcut and use the EBM calculator on our website and CD which allows us to convert an OR to an NNT at the click of a button (www.cebm.utoronto.ca). We interpret the NNTs and NNHs derived from SRs in the same way as we would for individual trials.

In the beta-blocker example, the risk of non-fatal MI was decreased [NNT 64 (49 to 107)] with use of beta-blockers as was the risk of myocardial ischemia [NNT 17 (14 to 22)]. However, there was a trend for increased all-cause mortality and cardiovascular mortality in patients who received beta-blockers. And, non-fatal stroke was increased in those who received beta blockers [NNH 282 (123 to 1208)]. Overall, this evidence suggests that there is no clear benefit to providing beta blockers to patients undergoing non-cardiac surgery.

Are the valid, important results of this systematic review applicable to our patient?

A SR provides an overall, average effect of therapy, which may be derived from a quite heterogeneous population. How do we apply this evidence to our individual patient? The same way we did it for individual trials – by

---

CARDS

Table 4.10 Formulae to convert odds ratios (ORs) and relative risks (RRs) to NNTs

For RR <1:
$$NNT = 1/(1 - RR) \times PEER$$
For RR >1:
$$NNT = 1/(RR - 1) \times PEER$$
For OR <1:
$$NNT = 1 - [PEER \times (1 - OR)]/(1 - PEER) \times (PEER) \times (1 - OR)$$
For OR >1:
$$NNT = 1 + [PEER \times (OR - 1)]/(1 - PEER) \times (PEER) \times (OR - 1)$$

Table 4.11 Translating odds ratios (ORs) to NNTs when OR<1

Patient expected event rate (PEER)	For odds ratio LESS than 1						
	0.9	0.8	0.7	0.6	0.5	0.4	0.3
0.05	209[a]	104	69	52	41	34	29[b]
0.10	110	54	36	27	21	18	15
0.20	61	30	20	14	11	10	8
0.30	46	22	14	10	8	7	5
0.40	40	19	12	9	7	6	4
0.50	38	18	11	8	6	5	4
0.70	44	20	13	9	6	5	4
0.90	101[c]	46	27	18	12	9	4[d]

[a]The relative risk reduction (RRR) here is 10%.
[b]The RRR here is 49%.
[c]The RRR here is 1%.
[d]The RRR here is 9%.

applying the guides for applicability listed in Table 4.13. One advantage that SRs have over most randomized trials is that the former may provide precise information on subgroups which can help us to individualize the evidence to our own patients. To do this, we need to remind ourselves of the cautions about subgroups we've summarized in Table 4.7.

Table 4.12 Translating odds ratios (ORs) to NNTs when OR>1

Patient expected event rate (PEER)	For odds ratio GREATER than 1						
	1.1	1.25	1.5	1.75	2	2.25	2.5
0.05	212	86	44	30	23	18	16
0.10	113	46	24	16	13	10	9
0.20	64	27	14	10	8	7	6
0.30	50	21	11	8	7	6	5
0.40	44	19	10	8	6	5	5
0.50	42	18	10	8	6	6	5
0.70	51	23	13	10	9	8	7
0.90	121	55	33	25	22	19	18

The numbers in the body of the table are the NNTs for the corresponding ORs at that particular PEER. This table applies both when a good outcome is increased by therapy and when a side-effect is caused by therapy.
(Adapted from John Geddes, pers comm 1999.)

CARDS

> Table 4.13   Is this valid and important evidence from a systematic review applicable to our patient?
>
> 1. Is our patient so different from those in the study that its results cannot apply?
> 2. Is the treatment feasible in our setting?
> 3. What are our patient's potential benefits and harms from the therapy?
> 4. What are our patient's values and expectations for both the outcome we are trying to prevent and the adverse effects we may cause?

Another advantage that systematic reviews have over individual trials is the ability to report on all important outcomes. For example, most trials do not have sufficient numbers of events (or duration of follow-up) to report on risk of adverse events of therapies. Systematic reviews can provide this information which can be helpful for us as we're considering risks and benefits of therapy with our patients.

> The high surgical risk subgroup had a 63% reduction in odds of all cause mortality and a 44% reduction in odds of non-fatal MI. However, there were too few events to provide definitive evidence of benefit for this subgroup of patients.

Further reading about systematic reviews

Egger M, Smith GD, Altman DG. *Systematic reviews in health care.* London: BMJ Books; 2001.

Haynes RB, Sackett DL, Guyatt G, et al. *Clinical epidemiology: How to do clinical practice research.* Philadelphia: Lippincott Williams & Wilkins; 2006.

Guyatt G, Rennie D, Meade M, et al., eds. *Users' guides to the medical literature. A manual for evidence-based clinical practice.* Chicago: AMA Press; 2008.

Practicing EBM in real-time: Using pre-appraised vidence

Often, tracking down and appraising the primary literature takes time that we can't afford during clinical practice and instead we can try to find high-quality pre-appraised evidence (as described in Ch. 2). For example, we could look for an answer to our question about dementia management with risperidone in *Clinical Evidence* (CE). (As mentioned in Ch. 2, CE (www.clinicalevidence.org) uses explicit, rigorous methods to retrieve, appraise, summarize and update relevant evidence.) In less than 30 seconds, we are able to find a relevant section in CE describing the evidence for risperidone (Figure 4.8). It outlines that its use is associated with increased risk of stroke and death and that alternate

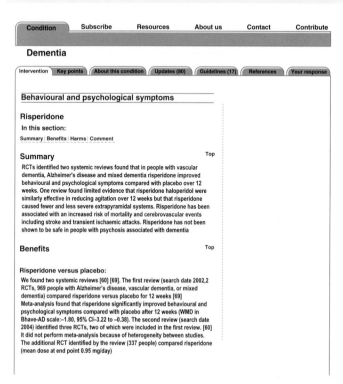

| Condition | Subscribe | Resources | About us | Contact | Contribute |

Dementia

| Intervention | Key points | About this condition | Updates (80) | Guidelines (17) | References | Your response |

Behavioural and psychological symptoms

Risperidone

In this section:

Summary | Benefits | Harms | Comment

Summary   Top

RCTs identified two systemic reviews found that in people with vascular dementia, Alzheimer's disease and mixed dementia risperidone improved behavioural and psychological symptoms compared with placebo over 12 weeks. One review found limited evidence that risperidone haloperidol were similarly effective in reducing agitation over 12 weeks but that risperidone caused fewer and less severe extrapyramidal systems. Risperidone has been associated with an increased risk of mortality and cerebrovascular events including stroke and transient ischaemic attacks. Risperidone has not been shown to be safe in people with psychosis associated with dementia

Benefits   Top

Risperidone versus placebo:

We found two systemic reviews [60] [69]. The first review (search date 2002,2 RCTs, 969 people with Alzheimer's disease, vascular dementia, or mixed dementia) compared risperidone versus placebo for 12 weeks [69]
Meta-analysis found that risperidone significantly improved behavioural and psychological symptoms compared with placebo after 12 weeks (WMD in Bhave-AD scale:–1.80, 95% CI–3.22 to –0.38). The second review (search date 2004) identified three RCTs, two of which were included in the first review. [60] It did not perform meta-analysis because of heterogeneity between studies. The additional RCT identified by the review (337 people) compared risperidone (mean dose at end point 0.95 mg/day)

4

Figure 4.8 *Clinical Evidence* screenshot. Risperidone.

---

strategies for behavior modification should be tried if possible. The benefits and harms of therapy and the CER, EER and OR are provided. Using this pre-appraised evidence, we can obtain the answer to our clinical question in less than 30 seconds, making it feasible to practice EBM in real-time at the bedside! Access to this resource can be arranged for a limited time so that you can try this search yourself.

Practicing EBM in real-time: pre-appraised literature for patients

---

Boots WebMD is a website that provides high quality information for patients. Searching on risperidone, we retrieve a synopsis of the evidence which highlights concerns about the risk of stroke and death

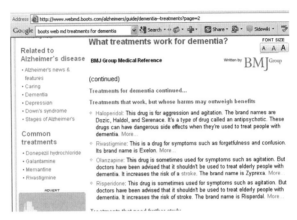

Figure 4.9 Boots WebMD screenshot. Information for our patient to review. Accessed 19 August 2010. Content written by and reproduced with permission of BMJ Group, screenshot reproduced with permission of Boots WebMD.

with its use and references that our patient may want to review (Figure 4.9). This material is based on the evidence reviewed for *Clinical Evidence*. It is freely available and something we can point our patients to.

A few words on qualitative literature

In this book, we've focused primarily on searching for and apprais-ing quantitative literature. Qualitative research may provide us with some guidance in deciding whether we can apply the findings from quantitative studies to our patients. Qualitative research can help us to understand clinical phenomena with emphasis on understanding the experiences and values of our patients. For example, returning to our patient described at the beginning of this chapter, we might want to look for studies that describe the experiences and feelings of patients like him who have taken antipsychotics or we might want to explore literature describing why patients might not comply with therapy. Or, we might want to explore the experiences of families towards aggressive behavior by their loved one who is affected with dementia.

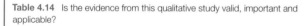

Table 4.14 Is the evidence from this qualitative study valid, important and applicable?
Are the results of this qualitative study valid? 1. Was the selection of participants explicit and appropriate? 2. Were the methods for data collection and analysis explicit and appropriate? Are the results of this valid qualitative study important? 1. Are the results impressive? Are the valid and important results of this qualitative study applicable to my patient? 1. Do these same phenomena apply to my patient?

The field of qualitative research has an extensive history in the social sciences but its exploration and development are relatively new to clinical medicine. We don't consider ourselves experts in this area and suggest that you take a look at the references we've included at the end of this section. We've included some guides in Table 4.14 that might be useful for evaluating the validity, importance and applicability of a qualitative study.

Are the results of this qualitative study valid?

1. Was the selection of participants explicit and appropriate?

We'd like to find that the authors included an appropriate spectrum of patients – by appropriate we mean that they represent the population that we are interested in and who are relevant to the study question. Random sampling of participants is usually not done and instead purposive sampling is used whereby the investigators explicitly select individuals who meet their specific criteria to reflect the experience they are assessing. For example, in a recent study evaluating the perceptions and experiences of clinician scientists with mentorship, rather than randomly sampling a group of academic physicians, investigators used purposive sampling to identify relevant clinicians.[21] Population Health and Clinician Investigators with MD degrees who obtained academic career support funding between 1996 and 2006 from the Alberta Heritage Foundation for Medical Research (AHFMR) were identified.

Stratified purposive sampling was used to ensure inclusion of participants from *both* Faculties of Medicine within Alberta, Canada and from both genders.

2. Were the methods used for data collection and analysis explicit and appropriate?

There are many different methods for collecting and analyzing data in a qualitative study and we need to ensure that the methods are explicitly outlined. We suggest you refer to some of the references mentioned at the end of this section to learn more about these methods. But, there are a few questions that you can start with. Did the investigators use direct observation (or audiotapes)? Did they conduct individual face-to-face interviews or focus groups? Was a text analysis used? Did the authors develop a conceptual framework and use the collected data to challenge and refine this framework in an iterative fashion? For example, in the recent mentorship study, the authors used a grounded theory approach and developed a conceptual framework using data from initial interviews. They subsequently used the data from a series of semi-structured interviews to challenge this framework and sampling of participants continued until saturation was achieved – by this we mean no new themes were raised by the participants. The authors used investigator triangulation whereby two or more investigators analyzed the data independently. Unlike quantitative research, where we try to find articles that describe blinded outcome assessors, blinding may not always be appropriate in qualitative research because it can limit the investigator's ability to interpret the data. Triangulation of source material can also occur; for example, interviews could be completed as well as field observations or document analysis.

Are the valid results of this qualitative study important?

1. Are the results impressive?

Does the report provide sufficient detail for us to obtain a clear picture of the phenomena described? Usually the results are presented narratively with relevant examples and quotes included to highlight themes. Sometimes authors include a quantitative component to outline dominant themes and demographic details. We include a sample from the mentorship study below.

Experience with mentorship

All participants believed good mentorship[21] to be vital to career success. The majority of participants experienced good mentoring. Nine mentee participants described difficulties with mentorship, including lack of mentorship, having research stolen by their mentor, or perceived competition with their mentor. They believed that these difficulties impacted on their career progress and productivity. One mentee stated: *"I don't know if I would perceive much mentoring during the time I have been on faculty."* Similarly, another mentee stated: *"I felt that I could have had more help than actually received."* A third mentee mentioned: *"I had a mentor who really didn't discuss things with me, was not interested in spending time on actually discussing issues, and was far too different from me to actually approach them with problems."*

Are the valid, important results of this qualitative study applicable to our patient?

1. Do we think these same phenomena apply to our patient/participant?

Does this paper describe patients similar to our own and do the phenomena described seem relevant to our patient? Ideally, the paper should provide sufficient information to allow us to determine if our patient is similar to those included in the study.

4

Further reading about individual randomized trials and qualitative studies

Guyatt G, Rennie D, Meade M, et al., eds. *Users' guides to the medical literature. A manual for evidence-based clinical practice.* Chicago: AMA Press; 2008.

Creswell JW. *Qualitative inquiry and research design.* London: Sage; 1998.

Adherence

Once our patient embarks on a chosen treatment, everything we and the patient have invested in diagnosis, critical appraisal, and individualizing the benefits and risks of therapy comes to nothing if the patient can't or won't follow his regimen of medication taking, diet, exercise, and the like. We call this patient behavior "adherence", and stress that our use of the term carries no implications about imperialistic clinicians or submissive patients. Briefly, adherence is a major problem in healthcare. Usual adherence is about 50% for both short- and long-term treatments (with a range of 0–100+++% and considerable variation within patients from week to week). The causes for low adherence rates are often not the ones we might think: age, sex, race, intelligence and education are not important. On the other hand, long waiting times, high cost, long duration and high complexity of treatments all lead to poor adherence. We should look for it any time a patient fails to reach a treatment goal (and especially before we increase a dose or add another drug). Irregular appointment keeping is a major clue, and a positive response to a single question, e.g., "Have you missed any pills in the past week?", when asked in a non-threatening way, generates a likelihood ratio (LR+) of 4.3 (see later for a discussion of likelihood ratios) for poor adherence (and an LR– of 0.5). If uncertainty persists, we can employ more expensive methods such as counting pills, checking prescription databases, measuring drug levels in body fluids, and providing special pill containers that keep a time record of dosing.

Our objective in detecting low adherence is to offer our patients strategies that might help them to adhere to therapy (but before doing so we should rethink the regimen and convince ourselves that it really is worth following!). Several adherence-improving strategies have been validated in randomized trials, but none leads to huge improvements. For short-term treatments they comprise exact instructions, preferably backed up by written information. For long-term care they include complex (and sometimes expensive) combinations of greater attention and supervision: more convenient care, information on the exact regimen (but not a detailed explanation of the disease, unless the patient wants one), counseling, reminders, self-monitoring, reinforcement, and family therapy.

Further reading about adherence

Haynes RB, Ackloo E, Sahota N, et al. Interventions for enhancing medication adherence. *Cochrane Database Syst Rev.* 2007;(1) CD000011.

Simel D, Rennie D. *Rational clinical examination: evidence-based clinical diagnosis.* Chicago: McGraw Hill; 2009.

Reports of clinical decision analyses

Occasionally, when we are attempting to answer a question about therapy, the results of our search will yield a clinical decision analysis (CDA). A CDA applies explicit, quantitative methods to compare the likely consequences of pursuing different treatment strategies and integrates the risks of benefit and harm associated with the various treatment options with values associated with the treatments and with potential outcomes. A CDA starts with a diagram called a "decision tree", which illustrates the target disorder, the alternative treatment strategies and their possible outcomes. A simple example is shown in Figure 4.10, which looks at the possible strategies for the management of atrial fibrillation, including anticoagulation, antiplatelet therapy, no antithrombotic prophylaxis, electrical and chemical cardioversion. The point at which a treatment decision is made is marked with a box. The possible outcomes that arise from the treatment strategies follow this decision node and are preceded by circles, called "chance nodes". The probabilities for each of these events are estimated from the literature (hopefully with a modicum of accuracy!) or occasionally from the clinician's clinical expertise. Triangles are placed at the end of each outcome branch and the patient's utility for each outcome is placed here. A utility is the measure of a person's preference for a health state and is usually expressed as a decimal from 0 to 1. Typically, perfect health is assigned a value of 1 and death is assigned a value of 0, although there are some outcomes that patients may think are worse than death and the scale may need to be extended below 0. Formal methods should be used to elicit utilities including the standard gamble and time trade-off techniques. Sometimes CDAs may use life-years, quality-adjusted life-years (or QALYs, where a year in a higher-quality health state contributes more to the outcome than a year in a poor-quality health state), or cases of disease or complications that are prevented. The utility of each outcome is multiplied by the probability that it will occur and this is summed for each chance node in the treatment branch to generate an average utility for that branch of the tree. The "winning" strategy, and preferred course of clinical action, is the one that leads to the highest utility. Note that this figure outlines a very simple tree – we could make it fancy and include the possibility of patients experiencing more than one outcome or health state.

While on clinical services, we've encountered an insurmountable time barrier to their use (and as mentioned, in discussions with our colleagues with significant expertise in this area, few are able to tackle them in real-time). To be done right, they have to generate and integrate probabilities and patient utilities for all pertinent outcomes, and particularize these probabilities and utilities to a specific patient. The result is elegant, and we sometimes wish we could do it for all our patients, but the process takes us an average of 3 days to complete just one simple tree. We've opted to use the more rough-and-ready but humanly feasible approaches

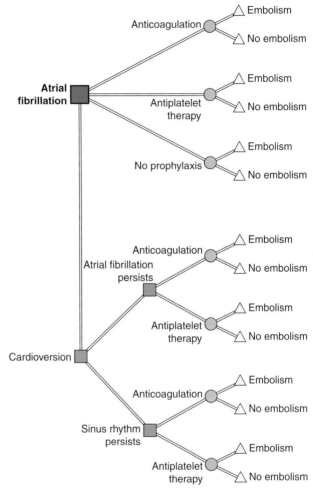

Figure 4.10 A simple decision tree.

for integrating evidence and patients' values such as the LHH. We don't consider ourselves experts at CDA and if you are interested in reading more about how to do them, check out the references at the end of this section. Typically, CDAs are most useful in policy decisions.

But even if we don't do CDAs, we sometimes read reports of them, and the rest of this section will briefly describe how we decide whether they are valid, important, and applicable to a patient. The guides that we use to do this follow.

Are the results of this CDA valid?

The CDA should include all the treatment strategies and the full range of outcomes (both good and bad) that we (and our patients) think are important (Table 4.15). For example, if we are interested in looking at a CDA that might help us determine the best management of patients with non-valvular atrial fibrillation and the CDA we find doesn't include aspirin as an alternative treatment to anticoagulants, we should be skeptical about its usefulness (since both work, albeit to different degrees). A CDA should explicitly describe a comprehensive, systematic process that was used to identify, select and combine the best external evidence into probabilities for all the important clinical outcomes. There may be some uncertainty around a probability estimate and the authors should specify a range; this may come from the range of values from different studies or from a 95% CI from a single study or systematic review. The methods that were used to assess the evidence for validity should also be included in the study. If a systematic review was not found to provide an estimate of the probability, were the results of the studies that were found combined in some sensible way? Finally, some investigators may use expert opinion to generate probability estimates, if these aren't available in the clinical literature, and these estimates won't be as valid as those obtained from evidence-based sources. In this case, it would be particularly important to do a sensitivity analysis to determine the impact of varying these estimates on the decision.

Were the utilities obtained in an explicit and sensible way from valid sources? Ideally, utilities are measured in patients using valid, standardized methods such as the standard gamble or time trade-off techniques. Occasionally, investigators will use values already present

Table 4.15 Is this evidence from a CDA valid?
1. Were all important therapeutic alternatives (including no treatment) and outcomes included?
2. Are the probabilities of the outcomes valid and credible?
3. Are the utilities of the outcomes valid and credible?

CARDS

in the clinical literature or values obtained by "consensus opinion" from experts. These latter two methods are not nearly as credible as measuring utilities directly in appropriate patients.

Ideally, in a high-quality CDA, the investigators should "discount" future events. For example, most people wouldn't trade a year of perfect health now for one 20 years in the future (we usually value the present greater than the future). Discounting the utility will take this into account.

If we think the CDA has satisfied all of the above criteria, we move on to considering whether the results of this CDA are important. If it doesn't satisfy the criteria, we'll have to go back to our search.

Are the valid results of this CDA important?

Was there a clear "winner" in this CDA, so that one course of action clearly led to a higher average utility? Surprisingly, experts in this area often conclude that average gains in QALYs of as little as 2 months are worth pursuing (especially when their CIs are big, so some patients enjoy really big gains in QALYs). On the other hand, gains of a few days to a few weeks are usually considered "toss-ups", in which both courses of action lead to identical outcomes and there is nothing to choose between them (Table 4.16).

Before accepting the results of a positive CDA we need to make sure it determined whether clinically sensible changes in probabilities or utilities altered its conclusion. If this "sensitivity analysis" generated no switch in the designation of the preferred treatment, it is a robust analysis. If, on the other hand, the designation of the preferred treatment is sensitive to small changes in one or more probabilities or utilities, the results of the CDA are uncertain and it may not provide any important guidance for our patient and us.

Are the valid, important results of this CDA applicable to our patient?

Once we've decided that the conclusions of a CDA are both valid and important, we still need to decide whether we can apply it to our patient (Table 4.17). Are our patient's probabilities of the various outcomes included in the sensitivity analysis? If they lie outside the range tested,

CARDS

Table 4.16 Is this valid evidence from a CDA important?
1. Did one course of action lead to clinically important gains?
2. Was the same course of action preferred despite clinically sensible changes in probabilities and utilities?

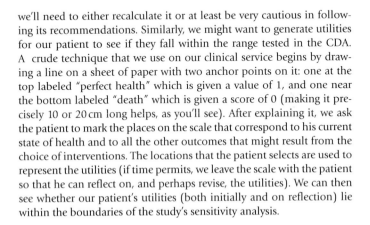

Table 4.17 Is this valid and important evidence from a CDA applicable to our patient?

1. Do the probabilities in this CDA apply to our patient?
2. Can our patient state his/her utilities in a stable, useable form?

CARDS

we'll need to either recalculate it or at least be very cautious in following its recommendations. Similarly, we might want to generate utilities for our patient to see if they fall within the range tested in the CDA. A crude technique that we use on our clinical service begins by drawing a line on a sheet of paper with two anchor points on it: one at the top labeled "perfect health" which is given a value of 1, and one near the bottom labeled "death" which is given a score of 0 (making it precisely 10 or 20 cm long helps, as you'll see). After explaining it, we ask the patient to mark the places on the scale that correspond to his current state of health and to all the other outcomes that might result from the choice of interventions. The locations that the patient selects are used to represent the utilities (if time permits, we leave the scale with the patient so that he can reflect on, and perhaps revise, the utilities). We can then see whether our patient's utilities (both initially and on reflection) lie within the boundaries of the study's sensitivity analysis.

Further reading about clinical decision analysis

Guyatt G, Rennie D, Meade M, et al., eds. *Users' guides to the medical literature. A manual for evidence-based clinical practice.* Chicago: AMA press; 2008.

Hunink M, Glasziou P, Siegel J, et al. *Decision making in health and medicine: integrating evidence and values.* Cambridge: Cambridge University Press; 2001.

Reports of economic analyses

Sometimes our search for an answer to a therapeutic or other clinical question will yield an economic analysis that compares the costs and consequences of different management decisions. We warn you at the outset that economic analyses are difficult to interpret and often controversial (even among health economists!) and we won't pretend to describe all their nuances here (if you are interested in understanding them, we've suggested some additional resources at the end of this section). They are very demanding for their investigators, and for us readers as well. They are most useful in policy-making decisions. These analyses teach us to stop thinking about the costs of a new treatment in terms of dollars and cents/pounds and pence, and to start thinking about them in terms of the other things we can't do if we use our scarce resources to fund this new treatment. This "cost as sacrifice" is better known as "opportunity cost" and is a useful way of thinking in everyday practice, for example, when we internists "borrow" a bed from our surgical colleagues in order to admit a medical emergency tonight, the opportunity cost of our decision includes canceling tomorrow's elective surgery on the patient for whom the bed was reserved.

These papers are pretty tough to read and you might want to confine your initial searches to the evidence-based journals (such as *ACP Journal Club*), which not only provide a standard, clear format for reporting economic analyses but also provide expert commentaries. The following guides should help you decide whether an economic analysis is valid, important, and useful.

Are the results of this economic analysis valid?

We need to begin by remembering that economic analyses (Table 4.18) are about choices and must therefore ensure that the study included all the sensible, alternative courses of action (e.g., anticoagulation, antiplatelet therapy and cardioversion for patients with non-valvular atrial fibrillation, NVAF) rather than just one or two of them. If, for example, we found a report that only described the costs of antiplatelet therapy for patients with NVAF, that's an exercise in accounting, not economic analysis, and it wouldn't help us. A valid economic analysis also has to specify the point of view from which the costs and outcomes are being viewed. Did the authors specify if costs and consequences are evaluated from the perspective of the patient, hospital or local government? For example, a hospital might shy away from inpatient cardioversion in favor of discharging a NVAF patient on anticoagulants that would be paid for from the family physician's drug budget, whereas society as

CARDS

Table 4.18 Is this evidence from an economic analysis valid?

1. Are all well-defined courses of action compared?
2. Does it provide a specified view from which the costs and consequences are being viewed?
3. Does it cite comprehensive evidence on the efficacy of alternatives?
4. Does it identify all the costs and consequences we think it should and select credible and accurate measures of them?
5. Was the type of analysis appropriate for the question posed?

a whole would want the most cost-effective approach from an overall point of view.

Because economic analyses assume (rather than prove) that the alternative courses of action have highly predictable effects, we need to determine whether they cite and summarize solid evidence on the efficacy of alternatives (the same caution we must remember when reading a CDA). So, was an explicit and sensible process used to identify and appraise the evidence that would satisfy the criteria for validity displayed back in Table 4.1?

All the costs and effects of the treatment should be identified, and credible measures should have been made of all of them. The cost side here can be tricky, since we may want the report to include all the costs including direct costs (e.g., cost of medication, hospitalization) and indirect costs (e.g., time lost from work). Moreover, a high-quality economic analysis should also include (and explain!) discounting future costs and outcomes (to acknowledge the fact that a bird in the hand is worth two in next year's bush).

We need to consider if the type of analysis was appropriate for the question the investigators posed, and this isn't as hard as it sounds. If the question was: "Is there a cheaper (but equally effective) way to care for this patient?", the paper should ignore the outcomes and simply compare costs (a "cost minimization" analysis). If the question was "Which way of treating this patient gives the greatest health 'bang for the buck'?", the method of analysis is determined by the sorts of outcomes being compared. If outcomes are identical for all the treatment alternatives (say, whether it's cheaper to prevent embolic stroke in NVAF patients with aspirin or warfarin), the appropriate analysis is a "cost-effectiveness" analysis. If, however, the outcomes as well as the interventions differ ("Do we get a bigger 'bang for our buck' treating kids for leukemia or the elderly for Alzheimer dementia?"), the authors will have had to come up with some way of measuring these disparate outcomes with the same yardstick, and there are two of these. They could convert all outcomes into monetary values: a "cost–benefit" analysis. The challenge in cost–benefit analysis is setting monetary values: should they be earning power (in which case we treat the kids and warehouse the elderly) or can we put a value on life itself? No wonder that cost–benefit analysis lacks popularity. The other common yardstick for disparate outcomes is their social (rather than monetary) value: how do patients view their desirability compared with other outcomes (including perfect health and death and fates worse than death)? A shorthand economic term for these preferences is "utility", and utilities can be com-

4

bined with time to generate "quality-adjusted life-years" (QALYs) (e.g., 1 year in perfect health is judged equivalent to 3 years in a post-stroke state whose utility is only 0.3). The corresponding economic analysis is called "cost–utility" analysis.

If the economic analysis fails the above tests for validity, it's back to searching. If it passes, we can proceed to considering whether its valid results are important.

Are the valid results of this economic analysis important?

Specifically, are the resulting costs or cost/unit of health gained clinically significant? We need to consider whether the intervention will provide a benefit at an acceptable cost (Table 4.19). If it is a cost-minimization analysis, we should consider if the difference in cost is big enough to warrant switching to a cheaper one. For a cost-effectiveness analysis, is the difference in effectiveness great enough for us to want to spend the difference? If a cost–utility analysis was done, how do the QALYs generated from spending resources on this treatment compare with those that would result if we spent them in other ways? This comparison is made superficially easier by cost–utility "league tables".***

Are the valid, important results of this economic analysis applicable to our patient/practice?

As usual, we begin by considering whether our patient is so different from those included in the study that its results are not applicable (Table 4.20). We can do this by estimating our patient's probabilities of the various outcomes, and by asking the patient to generate the utilities for these outcomes. If these values fall within the ranges used in the analysis, we can be satisfied that the "effectiveness" results can be applied to our patient. Next we can consider whether the intervention would be

Table 4.19   Is this valid evidence from an economic analysis important?
1. Are the resulting costs or cost/unit of health gained clinically significant?
2. Did the results of this economic analysis change with sensible changes to costs and effectiveness?

***If you want to learn more about league tables, we'd suggest you take a look at: Mason J, Drummond M, Torrance G. Some guidelines on the use of cost-effectiveness league tables. BMJ 1993; 306: 570–2.

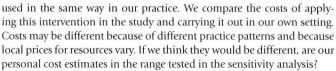

Table 4.20 Is this valid and important evidence from an economic analysis applicable to our patient?

1. Do the costs in the economic analysis apply in our setting?
2. Are the treatments likely to be effective in our setting?

used in the same way in our practice. We compare the costs of applying this intervention in the study and carrying it out in our own setting. Costs may be different because of different practice patterns and because local prices for resources vary. If we think they would be different, are our personal cost estimates in the range tested in the sensitivity analysis?

If the paper satisfies all of the above tests, we can celebrate. But if it fails any of them, it's back to the searching process!

Further reading about economic analysis

Guyatt G, Rennie D, Meade M, et al., eds. *Users' guides to the medical literature. A manual for evidence-based clinical practice.* Chicago: AMA press; 2008.

4

Reports of clinical practice guidelines

It seems that we cannot scan a journal or open our mail without finding information about a new clinical practice guideline. Clinical practice guidelines are systematically developed statements to help clinicians and patients with decisions about appropriate healthcare for specific clinical circumstances.[22] In addition, they may inform decisions made by policy-makers and managers. Huge amounts of time and money are being invested in their production, application and dissemination. Unfortunately, this often occurs with unnecessary duplication. We recently completed a search for guidelines on the management of heart failure and we were daunted when we retrieved over 1000 citations! And, not all guidelines are created equal! In a review of the quality of 217 drug therapy guidelines published in the 1990s, Graham and colleagues found that less than 15% met half or more of the 20 criteria assessing rigor of development.[23] Another challenge we encounter as clinicians is the overlap of guidelines and the lack of collaboration across guideline developers. For example, in our practice we have guidelines on assessment and management of hypertension, dyslipidemia, diabetes, stroke, cardiovascular disease, when ideally we need a single guideline that informs how to optimize vascular risk. The New Zealand Guidelines Group has led the world on trying to achieve this with their approach on optimizing vascular risk.[24] It is this type of approach that will enhance our ability to use the evidence from guidelines. This next section is to help busy clinicians to decide whether a guideline is worth using.

In a nutshell, if we're considering using a guideline, we should think of it as having two distinct components, as depicted in Table 4.21: first, the evidence summary ("here's the average effect of this intervention on the typical patient who accepts it") and second, the detailed instructions for applying that evidence to our patient. Then we should look at the two components individually. We apply our eye and nose to the first component, the evidence summary: our eye, to see if all the relevant evidence has been tracked down and graded for its validity; and our nose, to smell whether it has updated its review recently enough to still be fresh. Then we apply our ear to the second component to listen for any "killer Bs" (Table 4.22) in our neighborhood that would make its detailed instructions impossible to execute.

Valid guidelines create their evidence components from systematic reviews of all the relevant worldwide literature. The reviews that provide the evidence components for guidelines are "necessity-driven" and synthesize the best evidence (even if it is of shaky quality) that can be found to guide an urgent decision that has to be made. It necessarily follows

Table 4.21 The two components of practice guidelines

	Evidence component	Detailed instructional component
Bottom Line	"Here's the typical effect of this diagnostic/therapeutic/ preventive intervention on the typical patient."	"Here is exactly what to do to/ with this patient."
Underlying requirements	Validity, importance, up-to-datedness	Local relevance
Expertise required by those executing this component	Human biology, consumerism, clinical epidemiology, biostatistics, database searching	Clinical practice, patient values, current practice, local geography, local economics, local sociology, local politics, local traditions
Site where this component should be performed	National or international	Local
Form of output	Levels/Grade of evidence	Grades/Strength of recommendations, detailed instructions, flow charts, protocols

Table 4.22 The killer Bs

1. Is the *Burden* of illness (frequency in our community, or our patient's pre-test probability or expected event rate [PEER]) too low to warrant implementation?
2. Are the *Beliefs* of individual patients or communities about the value of the interventions or their consequences incompatible with the guideline?
3. Would the opportunity cost of implementing this guideline constitute a bad *Bargain* in the use of our energy or our community's resources?
4. Are the *Barriers* (geographic, organizational, traditional, authoritarian, legal, or behavioral) so high that it is not worth trying to overcome them?

that some recommendations in the second component of a guideline may be derived from evidence of high validity and others from evidence that is much more liable to error.

Are the results of this practice guideline valid?

Detailed guides for assessing the validity of practice guidelines have been developed using rigorous methodology and we'd suggest that you turn to these if you are particularly interested in this topic.[24] For example, the AGREE Collaboration[25] has developed an instrument for assessing validity of guidelines that includes items targeting six domains, such as scope and purpose, stakeholder involvement, rigor of development, clarity of presentation, applicability and editorial independence. Recently, AGREE has been updated and the collaboration is attempting to validate its use. In this section, we present a more basic version that you can use when appraising the validity of guidelines (Table 4.23).

Similar to high-quality CDAs and economic analyses, valid practice guidelines should include all relevant strategies (e.g., for diagnosis, screening, prognosis, and/or treatment) and the full range of outcomes (including the good and the bad) that are important. For example, a guideline by the Canadian Task Force for Preventive Health Care found that there was fair evidence of no benefit and good evidence of harm with routine teaching of self-breast examinations in women aged 40–69 years.[26] It was crucial for this guideline to include data not only on the impact of

Table 4.23 Guides for deciding whether a guideline is valid

1. Did its developers carry out a comprehensive, reproducible literature review within the past 12 months?
2. Is each of its recommendations both tagged by the level of evidence upon which it is based and linked to a specific citation?

this screening intervention on mortality, but also on the potential harm, including the emotional distress associated with unnecessary breast biopsies. Similarly a guideline on prostate cancer assessment and management should include the evidence around impact of screening with PSA. This step in guideline development highlights the need for relevant stakeholder engagement to ensure important outcomes are considered.

A valid practice guideline should also include a comprehensive, reproducible literature review. A comprehensive review needs to include all relevant articles in all relevant languages (e.g., some of the most important evidence for guidelines about family supports for patients with schizophrenia was published in Mandarin). Ideally, the guideline should describe explicitly the methods used to retrieve, appraise and synthesize the evidence.

Although we'd like to see therapy recommendations supported by evidence from systematic reviews of randomized trials, as we've discussed previously, such evidence might not always be available. It follows therefore that some guideline recommendations may be derived from high-quality evidence and others from evidence that is more prone to error. Because strength of evidence supporting guideline recommendations may vary, it is useful to have the strength of recommendations graded on the quality of evidence found. Accordingly, it is important that these different "levels" of evidence are acknowledged in tying the evidence to the clinical recommendations. Only in this way can we separate the really solid recommendations from the tenuous ones, and (if we want to appraise the evidence for ourselves) track them back to their sources. This need was recognized back in the 1970s by the Canadian Task Force on the Periodic Health Exam[27] and ever more sophisticated ways of describing and categorizing levels of evidence have followed.[28] In the present era, they have been an important element of at least some of the clinical texts on "evidence-based practice", in which each clinical recommendation is accompanied by an icon denoting the level of evidence that was employed in generating it. There are many levels of evidence that have been developed and are used by various guideline developers. This is another challenge for clinicians as we try to use guidelines – the need to become familiar with these different approaches to grading recommendations and what they mean. More recently, an international collaboration has developed GRADE which is an attempt to provide an explicit strategy for grading evidence and strength of recommendations.[29] GRADE classifies evidence into one of four levels: high, moderate, low and very low. Evidence can be downgraded or upgraded based on its quality. For example, a randomized trial might start off being high quality but on assessing it, it is found to be poor quality or have wide confidence intervals and is downgraded to low quality. The strength of recommendations is graded as strong or weak. When desirable effects of an intervention outweigh undesirable effects, a strong recommendation is made. Other factors that influence the strength of recommendation are uncertainty or variability in values and preferences or uncertainty about cost implications. There are pros and cons to the GRADE approach (as with all approaches) and training is required for using GRADE in guideline development.[30] Evidence to support that its use enhances implementation and decision-making by clinicians and patients is awaited. Table 4.24 has some examples of levels of evidence for therapy studies that we've found useful.

Table 4.24 Levels of evidence for therapy studies

Level of evidence	Therapy/prevention/etiology/harm
1a	Systematic review with homogeneity of RCTs[a]
1b	Individual RCT with narrow confidence interval[b]
1c	All or none[c]
2a	Systematic review (with homogeneity) of cohort studies
2b	Individual cohort study (including low-quality RCT; e.g., <80% follow-up)
3a	Systematic review (with homogeneity) of case–control study
3b	Individual case–control study
4	Case series (and poor quality cohort and case–control studies)[d]
5	Expert opinion without explicit critical appraisal, or based on physiology, bench research or "first principles"

[a]By homogeneity we mean that a systematic review is free of worrisome variations (heterogeneity) in the directions and degrees of results between individual studies. Not all systematic reviews with statistically significant heterogeneity are worrisome, and not all worrisome heterogeneity need be statistically significant.
[b]e.g., if the confidence interval excludes a clinically important benefit or harm.
[c]Met when all patients died before the Rx became available, but some now survive on it; or when some patients died before the Rx became available, but now none die on it.
[d]By poor-quality cohort study, we mean one that failed to clearly define comparison groups and/or failed to measure exposures and outcomes in the same (preferably blinded) objective way in both exposed and non-exposed individuals and/or failed to identify or appropriately control known confounders and/or failed to carry out a sufficiently long and complete follow-up of patients. By poor quality case–control study, we mean one that failed to clearly define comparison groups and/or failed to measure exposures and outcomes in the same blinded, objective way in both cases and controls and/or failed to identify or appropriately control known cofounders.

4

As you can see, satisfying these validity guides is a formidable task, and successful development of guidelines requires a combination of clinical, informational, and methodological skills, plus lots of time and money. For this reason, this first component of guideline development is best filled by a national or international collaboration of sufficient scope and size to not only carry out the systematic review but to update it as often as important new evidence appears on the scene.

Is this valid guideline applicable to my patient/practice/hospital/community?

The first (and most important) advice here is that if a guideline developed out of town tells us how to treat our patients in town, we should be very wary about its applicability. The ADAPTE group[31] has provided an approach for adapting guidelines to local context. They describe a 24-step process that can be used by decision-makers when considering how to modify a guideline, while trying to preserve the validity of the recommendations. Evidence supporting the validity of the use of this tool is in development.

While substantial advances have been made in the science of guideline development, less work has been done to enhance the implementability of guidelines. Often, recommendations lack sufficient information or clarity to allow clinicians, patients or other decision-makers to implement them. And guidelines are often complex and contain large numbers of recommendations with varying evidential support, health impact and feasibility of use in practice and decision-making. The GLIA tool is an initial attempt at meeting this challenge, but much work needs to be done to enhance the implementability of guidelines.[32] No tool assesses the overall ease with which a guideline can be implemented.

Good guideline development clearly separates the evidence component ("here's what you can expect to achieve in the typical patient who accepts this intervention") from the detailed recommendations component ("admit to an intensive care unit (ICU), carry out this ELISA test, order that treatment, monitor it minute by minute, and have your neurosurgeon examine the patient twice a day"). What if we have no ICU, can't afford ELISA tests, have to get special Ministry of Health permission to use the treatment, are caring for a patient whose next of kin doesn't like this sort of Rx, are chronically short-staffed, and our nearest neurosurgeon is 3 hours away?

The applicability of a guideline depends on the extent to which it is in harmony or conflicts with four local (sometimes patient-specific) factors, and these are summarized as the potential "killer Bs" of Table 4.22. Note that we are not implying that there are just four barriers to guideline implementation – indeed a systematic review of barriers to guideline implementation by physicians has identified more than 250![33] But we highlight some of the key barriers to consider as we're assessing a guideline. If you hear any of these 4 Bs buzzing in your ear when you consider the applicability of a guideline, be cautious. We should also bear in mind that barriers can become facilitators and we should also determine what facilitators to implementation might exist in our setting.

First, is the *Burden* of illness too low to warrant implementation? Is the target disorder rare in our area (e.g., malaria in northern Canada)? Or is the outcome we hope to detect or prevent unlikely in our patient (e.g., the pre-test probability for significant coronary stenosis in a young woman with nonanginal chest pain)? If so, implementing the guideline may not only be a waste of time and money, but it might also do more harm than good. Reflecting on this 'B' requires that we consider our patient's risk of the event and their unique circumstances as we do when assessing the applicability of any piece of evidence (Table 4.6).

Second, are our patients' or community's *Beliefs* about the values or utilities of the interventions themselves, or the benefits and harms they produce, compatible with the guideline's recommendations? Ideally, guidelines should include some mention of values, who assigned these values (patient derived or author derived) and whether they came from one source or many sources. The values assumed in a guideline, either explicitly or implicitly, may not match those in our patient or our community. Even if the values seem, on average, to be reasonable, we must avoid forcing them on individual patients because patients with identical risks may not have the same beliefs, values and preferences as those who are used or assumed in the guideline, and some may be quite averse to undergoing the recommended procedures. For example, early breast cancer patients with identical risks, given the same information about chemotherapy, make fundamentally different treatment decisions based on how they weigh the long-term benefit of reducing the risk of recurrence against the short-term harm of being nauseated and losing their hair.[34] Similarly, patients with severe angina at identical risk of coronary events, given the same information about treatment options, exhibit sharply contrasting treatment preferences because of the different values they place on the risks and benefits of surgery.[35] Although the average beliefs in a community are appropriate for deciding, for example, whether chemotherapy or surgery should be paid for with public funds, decisions for individual patients must reflect their own personal beliefs and preferences.

4

Third, would the opportunity cost of implementing this guideline (rather than some other one(s)) constitute a *Bargain* in the use of our energy or our community's resources? We need to remember that the cost of shortening the waiting list for surgery is lengthening that for family therapy. As decision-making of this sort gets decentralized, different communities are bound to make different economic decisions, and "healthcare by postal code" will and ought to occur, especially under democratic governments.

And finally, are there insurmountable *Barriers* to implementing the guideline in our patient (whose preferences indicate they'd be more likely to be harmed than helped by the intervention/investigation, or who would flatly refuse the investigations or intervention), or in our community? Barriers can be geographic (if the required interventions are not available locally); organizational (no stroke unit available in a hospital that admits patients with acute stroke); traditional ("But we've always done it the other way!"); authoritarian ("But you've always done it my way!"); legal (fear of litigation if a usual but useless practice is abandoned); or behavioral (when clinicians fail to apply the guideline or patients fail to take their medicine). There can be barriers at each stakeholder level – patients/public, healthcare providers, managers and policy-makers. Another classification system for barriers (and facilitators) to implementation refers to barriers pertaining to knowledge, attitudes and behaviours.[36] If there are major barriers, the potential benefits of implementing a guideline may not be worth the effort and resources (or opportunity costs) required to overcome them.

Changing our own, our colleagues', and our patients' behavior often requires much more than simply knowing what to do. If implementing a guideline requires changing behavior, we need to identify which barriers are operating and what we can do about them. Significant attention is now being paid to evaluate methods of overcoming these barriers including changing physician behavior. Indeed, the finding that providing evidence from clinical research is a necessary but not sufficient condition for the provision of optimal care has created interest in knowledge translation, the scientific study of the methods for closing the knowledge-to-practice gap and the analysis of barriers and facilitators inherent in the process.[37] We will describe this process more fully in a subsequent chapter.

So, in deciding whether a valid guideline is applicable to our patient/practice/hospital/community, we need to identify the 4 Bs that pertain to the guideline and decide whether they can be reconciled with its application (or whether we are facing one or more "killer Bs"). Note that none of these Bs (even when present as "killer Bs") has any effect on the validity of the evidence component of the guideline. Note also that the only people who are "experts" in the Bs are the patients and providers at the sharp edge of implementing the application component.

N-of-1 trials

You may not always be able to find a randomized trial or systematic review relevant to your patient. Traditionally, when faced with this dilemma, clinicians have conducted a "trial of therapy" during which we start our patient on a treatment and follow him to determine whether the symptoms improve or worsen while on treatment. Performing this standard trial of therapy may be misleading (and is prone to bias) for several reasons:

1. Some target disorders are self-limited and patients may get better on their own.

2. Both extreme lab values and clinical signs, if left untreated and reassessed later, often return to normal.

3. A placebo can lead to substantial improvement in symptoms.

4. Both our own and our patient's expectations about the success or failure of a treatment can bias conclusions about whether a treatment actually works.

5. Polite patients may exaggerate the effects of therapy.

If a treatment were used during any of the above situations, it would tend to appear efficacious, when in fact it was useless.

The N-of-1 trial applies the principles of rigorous clinical trial methodology to overcome these problems when trying to determine the best treatment for an individual patient. It randomizes time, and assigns the patient (using concealed randomization and hopefully blinding of the patient and clinician) active therapy or placebo at different times, so that the patient undergoes cycles of experimental and control treatment resulting in multiple crossovers to help both our patient and us to decide on the best therapy. It is employed when there is significant doubt about whether a treatment might be helpful in a particular patient, and is most successful when directed toward the control of symptoms or relapses resulting from a chronic disease. It's also helpful in determining whether symptoms may be

4

caused by a medication. Recently a group of investigators in Australia evaluated a study of N-of-1 trials of stimulants for children with attention deficit disorder. They found a successful strategy for completion of N-of-1 trials with support for individual clinicians by mail or telephone.[38]

Guides that we use in deciding whether or not to execute an N-of-1 trial are listed in Table 4.25. The crucial first step in this process is to have a discussion with the patient to determine his interest, willingness to participate, expectations of the treatment, and desired outcomes. Next we need to determine if formal ethics approval is required.[†††] If, after reviewing these guides, it is decided to do an N-of-1 trial, we use the following tactics (they are described in detail elsewhere):[‡‡‡]

• Come to agreement with our patient on the symptoms, signs or other manifestations of his target disorder that we want to improve, and set up a data collection method so that they can be recorded regularly.

Table 4.25 Guides for N-of-1 randomized trials

1. Is an N-of-1 trial indicated for our patient?
   • Is the effectiveness of the treatment really in doubt for our patient?
   • Will the treatment, if effective, be continued long term?
   • Is our patient willing and eager to collaborate in designing and carrying out an N-of-1 trial?
2. Is an N-of-1 trial feasible in our patient?
   • Does the treatment have a rapid onset?
   • Does the treatment cease to act soon after it is discontinued?
   • Is the optimal treatment duration feasible?
   • Can outcomes that are relevant and important to our patient be measured?
   • Can we establish sensible criteria for stopping the trial?
   • Can an unblinded run-in period be conducted?
3. Is an N-of-1 trial feasible in our practice setting?
   • Is there a pharmacist available to help?
   • Are strategies for interpreting the trial data in place?
4. Is the N-of-1 study ethical?
   • Is approval by our medical research ethics committee necessary?

[†††]At our institutions this is variable – in some places ethics and written consent is required and at others it isn't necessary because the objective is improved care for an individual patient who is our co-investigator.
[‡‡‡]Guyatt G, Rennie D. Users' guides to the medical literature. Chicago: AMA Press, 2002.

- Determine (in collaboration with a pharmacist and our patient) the active and comparison (usually placebo) treatments, treatment durations, and rules for stopping a treatment period.

- Set up pairs of treatment periods in which our patient receives the experimental therapy during one period and the placebo during the other (with the order of treatment randomized).

- If possible, both we and our patient remain blind to the treatment being given during any period, even when we examine the results at the end of the pair of periods. This means having a pharmacist independently prepare medications.

- Pairs of treatment periods are continued and analyzed until we decide to unblind the results and decide whether to continue the active therapy or abandon it.

- Monitor treatment targets regularly, using relevant outcomes decided upon by the patient and clinician.

Further reading about N-of-1 trials

Guyatt G, Sackett D, Adachi J, et al. A clinician's guide for conducting randomized trials in individual patients. *CMAJ*. 1998;139(6):497–503.

Guyatt G, Rennie D, Meade M, et al., eds. *Users' guides to the medical literature. A manual for evidence-based clinical practice*. Chicago: AMA press; 2008.

4

References

1. Ballard C, Hanney ML, Theodoulou M, et al. The dementia antipsychotic withdrawal trial (DART-AD): long-term follow-up of a randomized placebo-controlled trial. *Lancet Neurol*. 2009;8(2):151–157.

2. Schneider LS, Tariot PN, Dagerman K, et al. Effectiveness of atypical antipsychotic drugs in patients with Alzheimer's disease. *N Engl J Med*. 2006;355(15):1525–1538.

3. Stampfer MJ, Colditz GA. Estrogen replacement therapy and coronary heart disease: a quantitative assessment of the epidemiologic evidence. *Prev Med*. 1991;20(1):47–63.

4. Hulley S, Grady D, Bush T, et al. Randomized trial of estrogen plus progestin for secondary prevention of coronary heart disease in postmenopausal women. *JAMA*. 1998;280(7):605–613.

5. Rossouw JE, Anderson G, Prentice RL, et al. Risks and benefits of estrogen and progestin in healthy postmenopausal women: principal results from the Women's Health Initiative randomized controlled trial. *JAMA*. 2002;288(3):321–323.

6. The EC/IC Bypass Study Group. Failure of extracranial–intracranial arterial bypass to reduce the risk of ischemic stroke. Results of an international randomized trial. *N Engl J Med*. 1985;313(19):1191–1200.

7. Echt DS, Liebson PR, Mitchell LB, et al. Mortality and morbidity in patients receiving encainide, flecainide, or placebo. The Cardiac Arrhythmia Suppression Trial. *N Engl J Med*. 1991;324(12):781–788.

8. Moore T. *Deadly medicine: Why tens of thousands of heart patients died in America's worst drug disaster*. New York: Simon & Schuster; 1995.

9. Schultz KF, Grimes DA. Allocation concealment in randomized trials. *Lancet*. 2002;359(9306):614–618.

10. Online. Available: www.consort-statement.org/.

11. Deshauer D, Moher D, Fergusson D, et al. Selective serotonin reuptake inhibitors for unipolar depression: a systematic review of classic long-term randomized controlled trials. *CMAJ*. 2008;178(10):1293–1301.

12. Bassler D, Montori VM, Briel M, et al. Early stopping of randomized clinical trials for overt efficacy is problematic. *J Clin Epidemiol*. 2008;61(3):241–246.

13. Barnett HJ, Taylor DW, Eliaszew M, et al. Benefits of carotid endarterectomy in patients with symptomatic moderate or severe stenosis. *N Engl J Med*. 1998;339(20):1415–1425.

14. Devereaux PJ, Manns B, Ghali WH, et al. Physician interpretations and textbook definitions of blinding terminology in randomized control trials. *JAMA*. 2001;285(15):2000–2003.

15. Ferreira-Gonzalez I, Permanyer-Miralda G, Busse JW, et al. Methodologic discussions for using and interpreting composite endpoints are limited but still identify major concerns. *J Clin Epidemiol*. 2007;60(7):651–657.

16. The ADVANCE Collaborative Group. Intensive blood glucose control and vascular outcomes in patients with type 2 diabetes. *N Engl J Med*. 2008;358(24):2560–2572.

17. Montori VM, Malaga G. Intensive glucose control did not prevent important complications in type 2 diabetes. *ACP J Club*. 2008;149(3):6–7.

18. Hirsch C. Continued use of antipsychotic drugs increased long-term mortality in patients with Alzheimer disease. *ACP J Club*. 2009;150(12):JC6–JC8.

19. Bangalore S, Wetterslev J, Pranesh S, et al. Perioperative beta blockers in patients having non-cardiac surgery: a meta-analysis. *Lancet.* 2008;372(9654):1962–1976.

20. Liberati A, Altman DG, Tetzlaff J, et al. The PRISMA statement for reporting systematic reviews and meta-analyses of studies that evaluate health care interventions. *Ann Intern Med.* 2009;151(4):W65–W94.

21. Straus SE, Chatur F, Taylor M. Issues in the mentor–mentee relationship in academic medicine: A qualitative study. *Acad Med.* 2009;84(1):135–139.

22. Institute of Medicine. *Clinical practice guidelines: directions for a new program.* Washington DC: National Academy Press; 1990.

23. Graham ID, Beardall S, Carter AO, et al. What is the quality of drug therapy clinical practice guidelines in Canada? *CMAJ.* 2001;165(2):157–163.

24. Online. Available: www.nzgg.org.nz/guidelines/dsp_guideline_popup. cfm?guidelineID=35.

25. Online. Available: www.agreecollaborative.org.

26. Canadian Task Force for Preventive Health Care. Preventive health care, 2001 update. Should women be routinely taught breast self-examination to screen for breast cancer? *CMAJ.* 2001;164(13):1837–1846.

27. The Canadian Task Force on the Periodic Health Examination. The periodic health examination. *Can Med Assoc J.* 1979;121(9): 1193–1254.

28. Guyatt G, Rennie D, Meade M, et al., eds. *Users' guides to the medical literature. A manual for evidence-based clinical practice.* Chicago: AMA press; 2008.

29. Guyatt G, Oxman A, Vist G, et al, for the GRADE working group. GRADE: an emerging consensus on rating quality of evidence and strength of recommendations. *BMJ.* 2008;336(7650):924–926.

30. Brouwers MC, Somerfield MR, Browman GP. A for Effort: Learning from the application of the GRADE approach to cancer guideline development. *JCO.* 2008;26(7):1025–1026.

31. ADAPTE Group. *ADAPTE manual for guideline adaptation.* Online. Available: www.adapte.org May 27, 2008.

32. GLIA. Online. Available: http://gem.med.yale.edu/glia/login.htm; jsessionid=B6F586BB7B277D6C6BC2CFA4F746956B.

33. Cabana M, Rand C, Powe N, et al. Why don't physicians follow clinical practice guidelines? A framework for improvement. *JAMA.* 1999;282(15):1458–1465.

4

34. Levine MN, Gafni A, Markham B, et al. A bedside decision instrument to elicit a patient's preference concerning adjuvant chemotherapy for breast cancer. *Ann Intern Med*. 1992;117(1):53–58.

35. Nease RF, Kneeland T, O'Connor GT, et al. Variation in patient utilities for outcomes of the management of chronic stable angina: implications for clinical practice guidelines. *JAMA*. 1995;273(15):1185–1190.

36. Legare F, O'Connor AM, Graham ID, et al. Primary health care professionals' views on barriers and facilitators to the implementation of the Ottawa Decision Support Framework in practice. *Patient Educ Couns*. 2006;63(3):380–390.

37. Straus SE, Tetroe J, Graham ID. *Knowledge translation in health care*. Oxford: Wiley/Blackwell/BMJ Books; 2009.

38. Nikles CJ, Mitchell GK, Del Mar CB, et al. An n-of-1 trial service in clinical practice. *Pediatrics*. 2006;117(6):2040–2046.

5 Diagnosis and screening

Diagnosis is a complex and uncertain process, which is part intuition and part rationale. Before we look in detail at the rational "EBM" part of the process, we should look briefly at the wider process of diagnosis.

Experienced clinicians appear to combine two modes of thinking when engaged in clinical diagnosis.[1,2] In one mode, the clinician rapidly recognizes the patient's illness as a case of a familiar disorder; this is described as pattern recognition or non-analytic reasoning. In the second mode, the clinician uses features of the patient's illness to recall knowledge from memory and use it to analyze and deduce the correct diagnosis; this is termed analytic reasoning. Excellent clinicians employ both modes, using the faster, non-analytic method when it suffices, and slowing down to use the analytic approach when it is needed.[2] Within the analytic mode of reasoning, clinicians use several different approaches to analyzing patients' illness and in this chapter we'll focus on the probabilistic approach.

We can think of diagnosis as occurring in three stages[3]: initiation of diagnostic hypotheses ("I wonder if the patient has … "); refinement of the diagnosis by ruling out or narrowing possibilities ("It is not X or Y, but what type of infection could it be?"); and finally some confirmation of the final, most likely diagnosis ("We should do a biopsy to confirm this before treating."). These processes and some examples are illustrated in Figure 5.1. Initiation of the diagnosis includes gathering clinical findings and selecting patient-specific differential diagnoses for each potential diagnosis. Refining the diagnosis includes estimating the pretest probability for each potential disorder and defining the final diagnosis occurs when we are able to verify a diagnosis or cross a test/treat threshold, which is discussed later in this chapter.

In learning to be better diagnosticians we need to learn the many possible patterns, visual and non-visual, that we may encounter. With more than 10 000 possible diagnoses, that is a big task, and essential to the initiation phase – if we don't know of a diagnostic possibility, we cannot consider it. Each phase of the diagnostic process can be informed by relevant evidence. For example, evidence on the accuracy

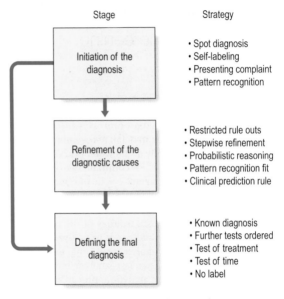

Stage	Strategy
Initiation of the diagnosis	• Spot diagnosis • Self-labeling • Presenting complaint • Pattern recognition
Refinement of the diagnostic causes	• Restricted rule outs • Stepwise refinement • Probabilistic reasoning • Pattern recognition fit • Clinical prediction rule
Defining the final diagnosis	• Known diagnosis • Further tests ordered • Test of treatment • Test of time • No label

Figure 5.1 Stages and strategies in the diagnostic process.[3]

of the clinical examination can help us with the initiation of diagnosis and research articles on disease probability can inform our attempts to define the pretest probability of various diagnoses. However, in the next phases, we will need to refine the diagnostic possibilities by using various diagnostic "tests" (including symptoms, signs, laboratory tests, and imaging), to refine and finally confirm the diagnosis. In this chapter, we will focus on three questions about these diagnostic "tests":

1. Is this evidence about the accuracy of a diagnostic test valid?

2. Does this (valid) evidence show that the test is useful at all?

3. How can I apply this valid, accurate diagnostic test to a specific patient?

After retrieving evidence about a test's accuracy, questions 1 and 2 suggest we need to decide if it's valid and important before we can apply the evidence to our individual patients. As with therapy, the order in which we consider validity and importance is not crucial, and depends on individual preference. Both should be done before applying the study results. Because the screening and early diagnosis of symptomless individuals have some similarities with, but also some crucial differences from, the diagnosis of sick ones, we'll close with a special section devoted to these acts at the interface of clinical medicine and public health. Tests may also be used for refining prognosis or for monitoring a disease, but we will not cover those in this chapter.

A central theme of this chapter is making sense of the uncertainties and inaccuracies in the process of diagnosis. Figure 5.2 shows the interpretation of the highly sensitive d-dimer for diagnosing deep vein thrombosis (DVT). The figure shows the post-test probabilities after positive (upper curve) and negative (lower curve) d-dimer results for the range of possible pre-test probabilities of DVT. The graph is based on the highly sensitive d-dimer having a *sensitivity* of 97.7% (that is, in those with DVT, 97.7% will have a positive result) and 46% specificity

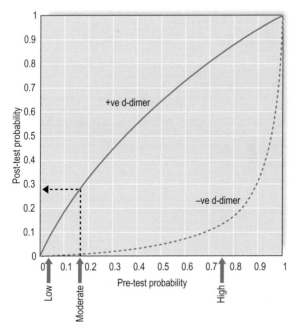

Figure 5.2 Probability revision graph showing a test's (d-dimer) impact on diagnostic uncertainty by how it changes the pre-test probability to the post-test probability (of DVT).

(that is, in those without DVT, 46% will have a negative result). The first question, on validity, asks if we can believe the information in the graph. The second question, on importance, asks if the results show clinically worthwhile shifts in uncertainty (the further apart the post-test curves, the larger this shift), and specifically whether the test helps to rule in or rule out the target disorder. The figure suggests that the highly sensitive d-dimer is helpful at ruling out over most of the pre-test range, but does not help to rule in. For example, for patients with a moderate (17%) chance of DVT based on the Well's score, the chance after a negative d-dimer is about 1%, but after a positive d-dimer, is still only about 28%. The third question means we need to understand how the test results might change our diagnostic uncertainty on application, not only for the patients in the study but more importantly, for a particular individual patient.

To further illustrate our discussion, we'll consider the following patient scenario.

Clinical scenario

Suppose that we're working up a patient with anemia and think that the probability that she has iron deficiency anemia is 50%, i.e. the odds are about 50:50 that it's due to iron deficiency. When we present the patient to our boss, she asks for an educational prescription to determine the usefulness of performing a serum ferritin on our patient as a means of detecting iron deficiency anemia.[4] By the time we've tracked down and studied the external evidence, our patient's serum ferritin comes back at 60 mmol/L. How should we put all this together?

Before looking at the scenario and our three questions, we should take a short detour through the land of "abnormality" so that what we might understand what could be meant by a normal or abnormal ferritin.

What is (ab)normal?

Most test reports will call some results "normal" and others "abnormal". There are at least six definitions of "normal" in common use (listed in Table 5.1). This chapter will focus on definition No. 5 ("diagnostic" normal) because we think that the first four have important flaws. The first two (the "Gaussian" and "percentile" definitions) focus just on the diagnostic test results in either a normal (the left-hand cluster in Fig. 5.3) or

Table 5.1 Six definitions of normal

1. *Gaussian:* the mean ± 2 standard deviations (SD) – this one assumes a normal distribution for all tests and results in all "abnormalities" having the same frequency.
2. *Percentile:* within the range, say of 5–95% – has the same basic defect as the Gaussian definition. Implies a specificity of 95% but with unknown sensitivity.
3. *Culturally desirable:* when "normal" is that which is preferred by society, the role of medicine gets confused.
4. *Risk factor:* carrying no additional risk of disease; nicely labels the outliers, but does changing a risk factor necessarily change risk?
5. *Diagnostic:* range of results beyond which target disorders become highly probable; the focus of this discussion.
6. *Therapeutic:* range of results beyond which treatment does more good than harm; means we have to keep up with advances in therapy!

5

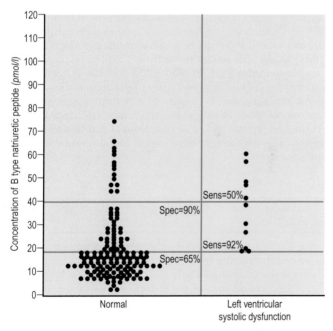

Figure 5.3 Distribution of B-type natriuretic peptide results in non-diseased (normal LVEF) and diseased (reduced LVEF) groups; two cutoffs are shown for 20 and 40 pmol/L.

an undifferentiated group of people (an unknown mix of the left and right clusters in Fig. 5.3), with no reference standard. They define the "normal range" on the basis of statistical properties (standard deviations or percentiles). They not only imply that all "abnormalities" occur at the same frequency, but suggest that if we perform more and more diagnostic tests on our patient, we are increasingly likely to find something "abnormal", thus leading to all sorts of inappropriate further testing.

The third definition of "normal" ("culturally desirable") represents the sorts of value judgment seen in fashion advertisements, and at the fringes of the "lifestyle" movement where medicine becomes confused with morality. The fourth ("risk factor") definition has the drawback that it "labels" or stigmatizes some patients regardless of whether we can intervene to lower their risk; this is a big problem with neonatal genetic testing and other screening maneuvers, as you'll learn in the concluding section of this chapter. The fifth ("diagnostic") definition is the one that we will focus on here, and we will show you how to work with it in the next section of this chapter. The final ("therapeutic") definition (does treating at and beyond this level do more good than harm?) is in part an outgrowth of the fourth ("risk factor") definition, but has the great clinical advantage that it changes with our knowledge of efficacy. Thus, the definition of normal blood pressure has changed radically over the past few decades as we have learned that treatment of progressively less pronounced elevations of blood pressure does more good than harm.

Is this evidence about the accuracy of a diagnostic test valid?

Having found a possibly useful article about a diagnostic test, how can we quickly critically appraise it for its proximity to the truth? The patients in the study should have undergone both the diagnostic test in question (say, an item of the history or physical examination, a blood test, etc.) and the reference (or "gold") standard (an autopsy or biopsy or other confirmatory "proof" that they do or do not have the target disorder). We can check that this was done well by asking some simple questions, and often we'll find their answers in the article's abstract. Table 5.2 lists these questions for individual reports, but we

Table 5.2	Is this evidence about a diagnostic test valid?

CARDS

1. *Representative:* Was the diagnostic test evaluated in an appropriate spectrum of patients (those in whom we would use it in practice)?
2. *Ascertainment:* Was the reference standard ascertained regardless of the diagnostic test result?
3. *Measurement:* Was there an independent, blind comparison with a reference standard?

(Fourth question to be considered for clusters of tests of clinical prediction rules)

4. Was the cluster of tests validated in a second, independent group of patients?

can also apply them to the interpretation of a systematic review of several different studies of the same diagnostic test for the same target disorder*.

1. Representative: Was the diagnostic test evaluated in an appropriate spectrum of patients (those in whom we would use it in practice)?

Did the report include patients with all the common presentations of the target disorder (including those with its early manifestations), and patients with other, commonly confused diagnoses? Studies that confine themselves to florid cases vs asymptomatic volunteers (a diagnostic "case–control" study) are useful only as a first crude check of the test, because when the diagnosis is obvious to the eye we don't need any diagnostic test. *(Note these study designs tend to overestimate test accuracy.)* The really useful articles will be set in the diagnostic dilemmas we face, and include patients with mild as well as severe; early as well as late cases of the target disorder; and among both treated and untreated individuals.

2. Ascertainment: Was the reference standard ascertained regardless of the diagnostic test's result?

When patients have a negative diagnostic test result, investigators are tempted to forego the reference standard, and when the latter is invasive

---

*As we'll stress throughout this book, systematic reviews provide us with the most valid and useful external evidence on just about any clinical question we can pose. They are still pretty rare for diagnostic tests and for this reason we'll describe them in their usual, therapeutic habitat, in Chapter 4. When applying Table 4.8 to diagnostic tests, simply substitute "diagnostic test" for "treatment" as you read. We look for the same things when considering the validity of diagnostic systematic reviews; specifically, was a comprehensive search completed, was a quality assessment of retrieved articles performed, and was there heterogeneity?

or risky (e.g., angiography) it may be wrong to carry it out on patients with negative test results. To overcome this, many investigators now employ a reference standard for proving that a patient does not have the target disorder which requires that the patient doesn't suffer any adverse health outcome during a long follow-up despite the absence of any definitive treatment (e.g., convincing evidence that a patient with clinically suspected deep vein thrombosis did not have this disorder would include no ill-effects during a prolonged follow-up despite the absence of anti-thrombotic therapy).

3. Measurement: Was there an independent, blind comparison with a reference ("gold") standard?[†]

In a study of test accuracy, we must determine if the test we're interested in was compared to an appropriate reference standard. Sometimes investigators have a difficult time coming up with clear-cut reference standards (e.g., for psychiatric disorders), and we'll want to give careful consideration to their arguments justifying the selection of their reference standard. Moreover, we caution you against the uncritical acceptance of reference standards, even when they are based on "expert" interpretations of biopsies; in a note in *Evidence-Based Medicine Journal*, Kenneth Fleming[5] reported that the degree of agreement over and above chance in reading breast, skin and liver biopsies is less than 50%! The results of one test should not be known to the people who are applying and interpreting the other (e.g., the pathologist interpreting the biopsy that comprises the reference standard for the target disorder should be "blind" to the result of the blood test that comprises the diagnostic test under study). In this way, investigators avoid the conscious and unconscious bias that might otherwise cause the reference standard to be "over-interpreted" when the diagnostic test is positive, and "under-interpreted" when it is negative. By independent, we mean that the completion of the reference test (or the test we're interested in) is not dependent on the results of the other.

[†]Note, to approximate the sequence of steps in the critical appraisal of therapy articles, we could consider the appraisal questions using the order **r**epresentativeness, **a**scertainment and **m**easurement. You'll notice that the first letters of these words produce the acronym, 'RAM' which some learners might find useful for remembering the appraisal questions. Alternatively, when considering the validity of reports of diagnostic test accuracy, others might find it easier to consider the most crucial question first; was there a comparison with an appropriate reference standard? If an appropriate reference standard was not used, we can toss the article without reading further, thereby becoming more efficient knowledge managers.

If the report we're reading fails one or more of these three tests, we'll need to consider whether it has a fatal flaw that renders its conclusions invalid. If so, it's back to more searching (either now or later; if we've already used up our time for this week, perhaps we can interest a colleague or trainee in taking this on as an "educational prescription"; see Ch. 1 if this term is new to you). On the other hand, if the report passes this initial scrutiny and we decide that we can believe its results, and we haven't already carried out the second critical appraisal step of deciding whether these results are important, then we can proceed to the next section.

Does this (valid) evidence demonstrate an important ability of this test to accurately distinguish patients who do and do not have a specific disorder?

Sensitivity, specificity and likelihood ratios

In deciding whether the evidence about a diagnostic test is important, we will focus on the accuracy of the test in distinguishing patients with and without the target disorder. We'll consider the ability of a valid test to change our minds from what we thought before the test (we'll call that the "pre-test" probability of some target disorder) to what we think afterwards (we'll call that the "post-test" probability of the target disorder). Diagnostic tests that produce big changes from pre-test to post-test probabilities are important and likely to be useful to us in our practice.

Returning to our clinical scenario, suppose further that, in filling our prescription we find a systematic review[6] of several studies of this diagnostic test (evaluated against the reference standard of a bone marrow stain for iron), decide that it is valid (based on the guides in Table 5.2), and find the results as shown in Table 5.3. The prevalence (or study pre-test probability) overall is 809/2,579 = 31%. For low ferritin (<65 mmol/L), the post-test probability of iron deficiency anemia among patients in the studies is $a/(a+b) = 731/1001 = 73\%$. This study post-test probability is known as the positive predictive value. For high ferritin (>65 mmol/L), the post-test probability of iron deficiency anemia among patients in the studies is $c/(c+d) = 78/1578 = 5\%$. This study post-test probability of 5%, means that the study probability of not having iron deficiency anemia after a negative result is 95%, which is known as the negative predictive value. So within the study, the uncertainty regarding iron deficiency has been shifted from the initial 31% to probabilities of either 73% or 5% – both appear to be clinically important shifts.

CARDS

Table 5.3 Results of a systematic review of serum ferritin as a diagnostic test for iron deficiency anemia

		Target disorder (iron deficiency anemia)		Totals
		Present	**Absent**	
Diagnostic test	Positive	731	270	1001
result (serum ferritin)	(<65 mmol/L)	a	b	a+b
	Negative	c	d	1578
	(≥65 mmol/L)	78	1500	c+d
Totals		a+c	b+d	a+b+c+d
		809	1770	2579

Data from: Guyatt GH, Oxman AD, Ali M, et al.[6]
Prevalence = (a+c)/(a+b+c+d) = 809/2579 = 31%.
Positive predictive value = a/(a+b) = 731/1001 = 73%.
Negative predictive value = d/(c+d) = 1500/1578 = 95%.
Sensitivity = a/(a+c) = 731/809 = 90%.
Specificity = d/(b+d) = 1500/1770 = 85%.
LR+ = sens/(1−spec) = 90%/15% = 6.
LR− = (1−sens)/spec = 10%/85% = 0.12.
Study pre-test odds = prevalence/(1−prevalence) = 31%/69% = 0.45.
Post-test odds = pre-test odds × likelihood ratio.
Post-test probability = post-test odds/(post-test odds + 1).

But we thought our patient's pre-test probability of iron deficiency anemia was greater than that in the study; in fact we estimated it to be 50% rather than the study's 31%. We could do a direct adjustment of the predictive values for the patient's different pre-test probability using the following equation:

patient post-test odds = study post-test odds ×
(patient pre-test odds / study pre-test odds)

which is analogous to the adjustment of a treatment trial's NNT for the patient's PEER. This is fine if you have the study in hand, but generally it is easier to derive some test accuracy measures – sensitivity and specificity, or the likelihood ratios – and apply these directly to the patient's individual pre-test probability. So let's look at these measures.

As you can see from Table 5.3, our patient's result (60 mmol/L) places her in the top row of the table, either in cell "a" or cell "b" You might note from Table 5.3 that 90% of patients with iron deficiency have serum ferritins in the same range as our patient [a/(a+c)]; that property, the proportion of patients with the target disorder who have positive test results, is called "sensitivity".

sensitivity = probability of a positive test given disease.

The complement of this proportion describes the proportion of patients who do not have the target disorder who have negative or normal test results, $d/(c+d)$, and is called specificity, that is:

specificity = probability of a negative test given non-disease.

(Note that non-disease here doesn't mean "no disease" but rather that it is not the target disease of the test).

You might also note that only 15% of patients with other causes of their anemia have results in the same range as our patient, which means that our patient's result would be about six times as likely (90%/15%) to be seen in someone with iron deficiency anemia as in someone without the condition; that ratio is called the "likelihood ratio" for a positive test result (LR+). The likelihood ratio positive is:

LR+ = probability of positive test result given disease /
      probability of positive test result given non-disease.

Since we thought ahead of time (before we had the result of the serum ferritin) that our patient's odds of iron deficiency were 50:50, that's called pre-test odds of 1:1. As you can see from the formulae towards the bottom of Table 5.3, we can multiply the pre-test odds of 1 by the likelihood ratio of 6 to get the post-test odds of iron deficiency anemia after the test $(1 \times 6 = 6)$; that's a post-test odds of 6:1 in favor of iron deficiency anemia. Since, like most clinicians, you may be more comfortable thinking in terms of probabilities than odds, the post-test odds of 6:1 converts (as you can see at the bottom of Table 5.3) to a post-test probability of $6/(6+1) = 6/7 = 86\%$. (To check yourself out on these calculations, try calculating the post-test probability for the same ferritin result for a patient who, like those in Table 5.3, has pre-test odds of 0.45[‡]; you'll know you did it right if you wind up with an answer for post-test probability that is identical to its equivalent, the positive predictive value.) Note that we could use the graph in Figure 5.4 (created with a program available on the accompanying CD) which allows us to determine the post-test probability, by drawing a line from the 50% pre-test probability to the post-test +ve line and across to the 86% post-test probability.

Once we know the sensitivity and specificity from a valid study, we can consider whether the test is useful and whether it can "rule out" or "rule in" the target disorder of interest.

5

[‡]The post-test odds are $0.45 \times 6 = 2.7$ and the post-test probability is $2.7/3.7 = 73\%$. Note that this is identical to the positive predictive value.

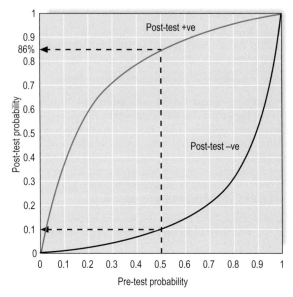

Figure 5.4 Probability revision graph. A test's impact on uncertainty: from pre-test to post-test probabilities.

Is the test useful at all?

As you might have guessed from our coin "test", if the sensitivity% and specificity% only add up to 100%, then the test is useless. It leaves the probabilities unchanged (and the post-test lines both lie on the diagonal of the pre-test/post-test graph). So for a test to be useful, the sensitivity% + specificity% − 100% (known as the Youden index) must be greater than zero (>0), and preferably be at least 50% (and ideally 100%!).

Can the test rule in or rule out?

Extremely high values (approaching 100%) of sensitivity and specificity with only modest specificity or sensitivity, respectively, can be useful. When a test has a very high sensitivity (such as the loss of retinal vein pulsation in increased intracranial pressure), a negative result (the presence of pulsation) effectively rules out the diagnosis (of raised intracranial pressure), and one of our clinical clerks suggested that we apply the mnemonic "SnNout" to such findings (when a sign has a

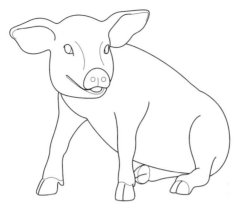

Figure 5.5 SnOut. When a sign has a high Sensitivity, a Negative result rules out the diagnosis.

high Sensitivity, a Negative result rules out the diagnosis) (Figure 5.5). Similarly, when a sign has a very high Specificity (such as the face of a child with Down's syndrome), a Positive result effectively rules in the diagnosis (of Down's); not surprisingly, our clinical clerks call such a finding a "SpPin" (when a sign has high Specificity, a Positive result rules in the diagnosis). Keep in mind that tests with extremely high sensitivity or specificity are rare. And, if you can find a perfect test that has 100% sensitivity and specificity, please let us know!

We can generate likelihood ratios directly or by reference to the sensitivity and specificity using the formulae in Table 5.3. The likelihood ratio for a positive test result:

LR+ = sensitivity/[1 − specificity]

and the likelihood ratio for a negative test result:

LR− = [1 − sensitivity]/specificity

(Finally, you might sometimes come across the diagnostic odds ratio, which is simply the LR+/LR−. If the diagnostic odds ratio is 1, then the Youden index will be 0). Table 5.4 illustrates the sensitivity, specificity, Youden index and likelihood ratios for some "tests" from the clinical examination. The first three are SnNouts and the next two are SpPins, but the last two rows are the most common – tests that are neither SpPins nor SnNouts, but they do give some information.

Table 5.4 Accuracy of selected tests from the physical examination

Test; condition	Sensitivity	Specificity	Youden index	LR+/LR−
Postural pulse increase >30/min; large blood loss	98	99	97	98/50
Brachio-radial delay; severe aortic stenosis	97	62	59	2.5/0.04
Dullness >10.5 cm from midsternal line; CTR >0.5	97	61	58	2.5/0.05
Diastolic BP <50 mmHg; moderate-to-severe aortic stenosis	30–50	98	38	20/0.6
Lachman sign; anterior cruciate ligament tear	48–96	90–99	66	17/0.2
Pulse >90 beats/min; hyperthyroidism	80	82	62	4.4/0.24
Dry mouth	85	58	43	2.0/0.3

All tests taken from McGee S. Evidence-Based physical diagnosis. 2nd edn. Philadelphia: Saunders, 2007.

Can I apply this valid, important diagnostic test to a specific patient?

Having found a valid systematic review or individual report about a diagnostic test, and having decided that its accuracy is sufficiently high to be useful, how do we apply it to our patient? To transfer the study results, adapt them to our patient's unique pre-test probability, and decide this would be clinically useful, there are three questions we should ask that are summarized in Table 5.5.

1. Is the diagnostic test available, affordable, accurate, and precise in our setting?

We obviously can't order a test that is not available. Even if it is available, we may want to check around to be sure that it's performed in a similar manner to the study, interpreted in a competent, reproducible fashion and that its potential consequences (see below) justify its cost. For example, some of us work on medical units at more than one hospital and have found that the labs at these different hospitals use different assays for assessing BNP – making the interpretation for the clinician

Table 5.5 Are the results of this diagnostic study applicable to my patient?

1. Is the diagnostic test available, affordable, accurate, and precise in our setting?
2. Can we generate a clinically sensible estimate of our patient's pre-test probability?
   a. From personal experience, prevalence statistics, practice databases, or primary studies
   b. Are the study patients similar to our own?
   c. Is it unlikely that the disease possibilities or probabilities have changed since this evidence was gathered?
3. Will the resulting post-test probabilities affect our management and help our patient?
   a. Could it move us across a test–treatment threshold?
   b. Would our patient be a willing partner in carrying it out?
   c. Would the consequences of the test help our patient reach his or her goals in all this?

more challenging. Moreover, diagnostic tests often behave differently among different subsets of patients, generating higher likelihood ratios in later stages of florid disease, and lower likelihood ratios in early, mild stages.

At least some diagnostic tests based on symptoms or signs lose power as patients move from primary care to secondary and tertiary care. Reference back to Table 5.3 can show you why. If patients are referred onward, in part because of symptoms, their primary care clinicians will be sending along patients in both cells "a" and "b", and subsequent evaluations of the accuracy of their symptoms will tend to show falling specificity due to the referral of patients with false-positive findings. If we think that any of these factors may be operating, we can try out what we judge to be clinically sensible variations in the likelihood ratios for the test result and see whether the results alter our post-test probabilities in a way that changes our diagnosis (the short-hand term for this sort of exploration is "sensitivity analysis").

2. Can we generate a clinically sensible estimate of our patient's pre-test probability?

This is a key topic, and deserves its own "section-within-a-section". As we said above, unless our patient is a close match with the study population, we'll need to "adjust" the study post-test probability to account for the pre-test probability in our patient. How can we estimate our patient's pre-test probability? We've used five different sources for this

151

vital information: clinical experience, regional or national prevalence statistics, practice databases, the original report we used for deciding on the accuracy and importance of the test, and studies devoted specifically to determining pre-test probabilities. Although the last is the ideal, we'll take each in turn.

First, we can recall our clinical experience with prior patients who presented with the same clinical problem, and back-track from their final diagnoses to their pre-test probabilities. While easily and quickly accessed, our memories are often distorted by our last patient, our most dramatic (or embarrassing) patient, our fear of missing a rare but treatable cause, and the like, so we use this source with caution.[§] If we're early in our careers, we may not have enough clinical experience to draw upon. Thus, while we always use our remembered cases, we need to learn to supplement them with other sources, unless we have the time and energy to document all of our diagnoses and generate our own database.

Second, we could turn to regional or national prevalence statistics on the frequencies of the target disorders in the general population or some subset of it. Estimates from these sources are only as good as the accuracy of their diagnoses, and although they can provide some guidance for "baseline" pre-test probabilities before taking symptoms into account (useful, say, for patients walking into a general practice), we may be more interested in pre-test probabilities in just those persons with a particular symptom.

Third, we could overcome the foregoing problems by tracking down local, regional or national practice databases that collect patients with the same clinical problem and report the frequency of disorders diagnosed in these patients. While some examples exist, such databases are mostly things of the future. As before, their usefulness will depend on the extent to which they use sensible diagnostic criteria and clear definitions of presenting symptoms.

Fourth, we could simply use the pre-test probabilities observed in the study we critically appraised for the accuracy and importance of the diagnostic test. If they really did sample the full spectrum of patients with the symptom or clinical problem (the second of our accuracy guides), we can extrapolate the pre-test probability from their study patients (or some subgroup of it) to our patient.

[§]If you want to read more about how our minds and memories can distort our clinical reasoning, start with: Kassirer JP, Kopelman RI. Cognitive errors in diagnosis: instantiation, classification and consequences. Am J Med 1989; 86 (4): 433–441.

Fifth and finally, we could track down a research report of a study expressly devoted to documenting pre-test probabilities for the array of diagnoses that present with a specific set of symptoms and signs similar to our patient. When done well, among patients closely similar to our patient, these studies provide the least biased source of pre-test probabilities for our use. Such studies are challenging to carry out, and one of us led the group who generated guides for their critical appraisal.[7] We've summarized these guides in Table 5.6. You'll see that most of them are already familiar to you, for they apply equally to reports of the accuracy and importance of diagnostic tests. We've provided examples of pre-test probabilities on our website (www.cebm.utoronto.ca).

3. Will the resulting post-test probabilities affect our management and help our patient?

There are three elements of the answer to this final question and we begin with the bottom line: Could its results move us across some threshold that would cause us to stop all further testing? Two thresholds should be borne in mind, as shown in Figure 5.6. First, if the diagnostic test was negative or generated a likelihood ratio down near 0.1, the post-test probability might become so low that we would abandon the diagnosis we were pursuing, and turn to other diagnostic possibilities. Put in terms of thresholds, this negative test result has moved us from above to below the "test threshold" in Figure 5.6 and we won't do any more tests for that diagnostic possibility. On the other hand, if the diagnostic test came back positive or generated a high likelihood ratio, the post-test probability might become so high that we would also abandon

Table 5.6 Guides for critically appraising a report about pre-test probabilities of disease

1. Is this evidence about pre-test probability valid?
   a. Did the study patients represent the full spectrum of those who present with this clinical problem?
   b. Were the criteria for each final diagnosis explicit and credible?
   c. Was the diagnostic work-up comprehensive and consistently applied?
   d. For initially undiagnosed patients, was follow-up sufficiently long and complete?
2. Is this evidence about pre-test probability important?
   a. What were the diagnoses and their probabilities?
   b. How precise were these estimates of disease probability?

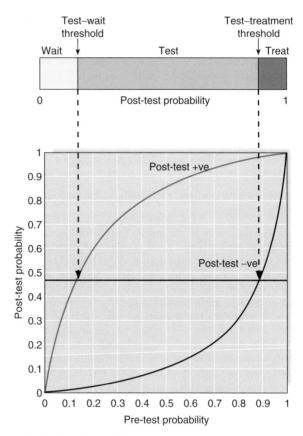

Figure 5.6 Test-treatment thresholds.

further testing because we've made our diagnosis and would now move to choosing the most appropriate therapy; in these terms, we've now crossed from below to above the "treatment threshold" in Figure 5.6.

It is only if our diagnostic test result leaves us stranded between the test and treatment thresholds that we would continue to pursue that initial diagnosis by performing other tests. Although there are some very fancy ways of calculating test–treatment thresholds from test accuracy and the risks and benefits of correct and incorrect diagnostic conclusions,** intuitive test–treatment thresholds are commonly used by experienced clinicians and are another example of individual clinical expertise. We suggest you look at several pre-test scenarios using a post-test probability graph (Figure 5.4) to get a feel of when the test results in clinically useful shifts in decisions.

We may not cross a test–treatment threshold until we've performed several different diagnostic tests, and here is where another nice property of the likelihood ratio comes into play: provided the tests are independent we can "chain" the likelihood ratios. The post-test odds that result after the first diagnostic test we apply, become the pre-test odds for our second diagnostic test. Hence, we can simply keep multiplying the running product by the likelihood ratio generated from the next test. For example, when a 45-year-old man walks into our office, his pre-test probability of >75% stenosis of one or more of his coronary arteries is about 6%. Suppose that he gives us a history of atypical chest pain (only two of the three symptoms of substernal chest discomfort, brought on by exertion, and relieved in less than 10 minutes by rest are present, generating a likelihood ratio of about 13) and that his exercise ECG reveals 2.2 mm of non-sloping ST-segment depression (generating a likelihood ratio of about 11). Then his post-test probability for coronary stenosis is his pre-test probability (converted into odds) times the product of the likelihood ratios generated from his history and exercise ECG, with the resulting post-test odds converted back to probabilities (through dividing by its value + 1), i.e.:

$$(0.06 / 0.94) \times 13 \times 11 = 9.13, \text{ and then } 913 / 1013 = 90\%.$$

The final result of these calculations is strictly accurate as long as the diagnostic tests being combined are "independent" (i.e. given the "true" condition, the accuracy of one test does not further depend on another test). However, some dependence is common, and means we tend to overestimate the informativeness of the multiple tests. Accordingly, we would want the calculated post-test probability at the end of this sequence to be comfortably above our treatment threshold before we would act upon it. This additional example of how likelihood ratios make lots of implicit diagnostic reasoning explicit is another argument in favor of seeking reports of overall likelihood ratios for sequences or clusters of diagnostic tests (see below).

**See the recommendations for additional reading or: Pauker SG, Kassirer JP. The threshold approach to clinical decision making. NEJM 1980; 302 (20): 1109.

We should have kept our patient informed as we worked our way through all the foregoing considerations, especially if we've concluded that the diagnostic test is worth considering. If we haven't yet done so, we certainly need to do so now. Every diagnostic test involves some invasion of privacy, and some are embarrassing, painful, or dangerous. We'll have to be sure that the patient is an informed, willing partner in the undertaking. In particular, they should be aware of the possibility of false-positive or false-negative outcomes so that this is not a surprise when they return to discuss the results. The ultimate question to ask about using any diagnostic test is whether its consequences (reassurance when negative, labeling and possibly generating awful diagnostic and prognostic news if positive, leading to further diagnostic tests and treatments, etc.) will help our patient achieve his or her goals of therapy. Included here are considerations of how subsequent interventions match clinical guidelines or restrictions on access to therapy designed to optimize the use of finite resources for all members of our society.

Multilevel likelihood ratios

The more extreme a test result is, the more persuasive it is. Although the dichotomized serum ferritin's sensitivity (90%) and specificity (85%) look impressive, expressing its accuracy with level-specific likelihood ratios reveals its even greater power and, in this particular example, shows how we can be misled by the restriction to just two levels (positive and negative) of the test result. Many test results, like serum ferritin, can be divided into several levels, and in the CAT (see Table 5.8) we show you a particularly useful way of dividing test results into five levels.

When this is done, we see how much more informative extreme ferritin results are. The LR for the "very positive" result is a huge 52, so that one extreme level of the test result can be shown to rule in the diagnosis, and in this case we can SpPin 59% (474/809) of the patients with iron deficiency anemia, despite the unimpressive sensitivity (59%) that would have been achieved if the ferritin results had been split just below this level. Likelihood ratios of 10 or more, when applied to pre-test probabilities of 33% or more (0.33/0.67 = pre-test odds of 0.5) will generate post-test probabilities of 5/6 = 83% or more.

Similarly, the other extreme level (>95) is a SnNout 75% (1332/1770) for those who do not have iron deficiency anemia (again despite a not-very-impressive specificity of 75%). Likelihood ratios of ≤0.1, when applied to pre-test probabilities of ≤33% (0.33/0.67 = pre-test odds of 0.5) will generate post-test probabilities of 0.05/1.05 = 5% or less. The two intermediate levels (moderately positive and moderately negative) can move a 50% prior probability (pre-test odds of 1:1) to the useful but not necessarily diagnostic post-test probabilities of 4.8/5.8 = 83% and 0.39/1.39 = 28%. And the indeterminate level ("neutral") in the middle (containing about 10% of both sorts of patients) can be seen to be uninformative, with a likelihood ratio of 1. When diagnostic test accuracy results are around 1.0, we've learned nothing by ordering them. To give you a better "feel" for this, the impact of different likelihood ratios on different pre-test probabilities are shown in Figure 5.7. We've provided additional examples of likelihood ratios on this book's website (www. cebm.utoronto.ca).

An easier way of manipulating all these calculations is the nomogram of Figure 5.8 (also provided in the pocket cards that come with this book). You can check out your understanding of this nomogram by using it to replicate the results of Table 5.3.

Now return to our patient with a pre-test probability for iron deficiency of 50% and a ferritin result of 60 mmol/L. To your surprise (we reckon!), our patient's test result generates an indeterminate likelihood ratio of

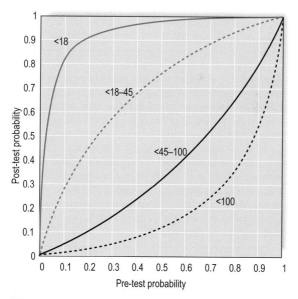

Figure 5.7 Different post-test probabilities for four ferritin results.

CARDS

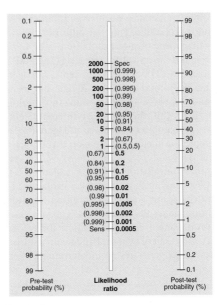

Figure 5.8 Likelihood ratio nomogram.

only 1, and the test which we thought might be very useful, based on the old sensitivity and specificity way of looking at things, really hasn't been helpful in moving us toward the diagnosis. We'll have to think about other tests (including perhaps the reference standard of a bone marrow examination) to sort out the patient's diagnosis.

More and more reports of diagnostic tests are providing multilevel likelihood ratios as measures of their accuracy. When their abstracts report only sensitivity and specificity, we can sometimes find a table with more levels and generate our own set of likelihood ratios; at other times we can find a scatterplot (of test results vs diagnoses) that is good enough for us to be able to split them into levels.

Multiple tests

Some reports of diagnostic tests go beyond even likelihood ratios, and one of their extensions deserves mention here. This extension considers multiple diagnostic tests as a cluster or sequence of tests for a given target disorder. These multiple results can be presented in different ways, either

Table 5.7 Examples of clinical prediction rules		
Prediction rule	**Sensitivity**	**Specificity**
Ottawa Ankle Rule[8]	99.6%	48%
ABCD rule for melanoma[9]	84%	56%
Well's DVT Rule[10]	Multilevel test	
ABCD rule for stroke prediction after TIA[11]	Multilevel test	

as clusters of positive/negative results or as multivariate scores, and in either case they can be ranked and handled just like other multilevel likelihood ratios. Some examples of common clinical prediction rules are given in Table 5.7.

When they perform (nearly) as well in a second, independent ("test") set of patients, we often refer to them as "clinical prediction guides" (CPGs). In appraising the validity of a study of a CPG, we need to consider a fourth question in addition to those above.

Was the cluster of tests validated in a second, independent group of patients?

Diagnostic tests are predictors, not explainers, of diagnoses. As a result, their initial evaluation cannot distinguish between real diagnostic accuracy for the target disorder and chance associations due to idiosyncrasies in the initial ("training" or "derivation") set of patients. This problem is compounded for clusters of diagnostic features (often called "clinical prediction guides"), where the large number of possible tests considered means we may overestimate the value of the few chosen in the CPG. The best indicator of accuracy in these situations is the demonstration of similar levels of accuracy when the test or cluster is evaluated in a second, independent (or "test") set of patients. If it performs well in this "test" set, we are reassured about its accuracy. If it performs poorly, we should look elsewhere. And if no "test set" study has been carried out, we'd be wise to reserve judgment. Clinical prediction guides are also used to help establish prognosis. Detailed appraisal guides for clinical prediction guides are available and we refer you to the textbooks mentioned at the end of this chapter for more information.

Practicing EBM in real-time

Clinical prediction guides often include several variables that we have to remember when trying to apply them to our patients. Several colleagues have attempted to make this easier and have provided interactive versions of clinical prediction guides available on websites (e.g., http://www.mssm.edu/medicine/general-medicine/ebm/). We've also provided some of these on the accompanying website.

TM

Learning and teaching with CATs

Now that we have invested precious time and energy into finding and critically appraising an article, it would be a shame not to summarize and keep track of it so that we (and others) can use it again in the future. The means invented by Stephane Sauve, Hui Lee, and Mike Farkouh, residents on Dave Sackett's clinical service several years ago, to accomplish this was to create a standardized one-page summary of the evidence organized as a "critically appraised topic", which they called a "CAT". A CAT begins with a declarative title and quickly states a clinical "bottom line" describing the clinical action that follows from the paper. To assist later updating of the CAT, the three- or four-part clinical question that started the process, and the search terms that were used to locate the paper are included in it. Next is a summary of the study methods and a table summarizing the key results. Any issues important to bear in mind when applying the CAT (such as rare adverse effects, costs, or unusual elements of the critical appraisal) are inserted beneath the results table. Now take a look at the CAT we generated for ferritin (Table 5.8).

Screening and case-finding

So far, this chapter has focused on making a diagnosis for sick patients who have come to us for help. They are asking us to diagnose their ills and to help them as best we can, and only charlatans guarantee them longer life at the initial encounter. This final section of the chapter focuses on making early diagnoses of pre-symptomatic disease among well individuals in the general public (we'll call that "screening") or among patients who have come to us for some other unrelated disorder (we'll call that "case-finding"). Individuals whom we might consider for screening and case-finding are not ill from the target disorders, so we are soliciting them with the promise (overt or covert) that they will live longer, or at least better, if they let us test them. Accordingly, the evidence we need about the validity of screening and case-finding goes beyond the accuracy of the test for early diagnosis; we need hard evidence that patients are better off, in the long run, when such early diagnosis is achieved.

Table 5.8 CAT: Ferritin can diagnose iron deficiency in the elderly

Clinical bottom line: Serum ferritin can be very useful in diagnosing iron deficiency anemia in the elderly.

Clinical scenario. 75-year-old retired schoolteacher (in for a check-up) found to have a Hb of 100, with an MCV of 80, a negative history and physical, and on no medications that are likely to suppress her marrow or cause a bleed. I think her probability of iron deficiency is 1 out of 2 or 50%.

Three-part question. In an elderly symptomless woman with mild anemia, would a serum ferritin help determine whether her bone marrow iron stores were depleted?

Search terms. Searching *ACP Journal Club* using the terms 'iron deficiency anemia' and 'ferritin', we find a study that appears to be of interest and that provides a link to an overview of this topic.

The study

Patients. Consecutive anemic patients in several inpatient and outpatient settings. Transfused patients excluded.

Target disorder and gold standard. Bone marrow, stained for iron.

Diagnostic test. Serum ferritin by radioimmunoassay.

Representative appropriate spectrum … ?	Can't tell
Standard applied regardless of test result … ?	Yes
Measurements: Blind … ?	Yes
Objective … ?	Probably

The evidence

	Present		Absent		
Test result	No.	Prop.	No.	Prop.	LR
<15	474	0.59	20	0.01	51.85
15–34	175	0.22	79	0.04	4.85
35–64	82	0.10	171	0.11	1.05
65–94	30	0.04	168	0.09	0.39
≥95	48	0.06	1332	0.75	0.08

Comments

1. For elderly patients with symptomless anemia, go to the CAT on anemia in the elderly to determine the yields from upper and lower GI investigations.
2. Lots of labs are very slow in returning ferritin requests.

Expiry date: …2010.

All screening and case-finding, at least in the short-run, harms some people. Early diagnosis is just that: people are "labeled" as having, or as being at high risk for developing, some pretty awful diseases (cancer of the breast, stroke, heart attack, and the like). And this labeling takes place months, years, or even decades before the awful diseases will become manifest as symptomatic illness (often in only a small portion of those who screen positive). Labeling hurts. For example, a cohort of working men studied both before and after they were labeled hypertensive displayed increased absenteeism, decreased psychological well-being, and progressive loss of income in comparison to their normotensive workmates (and these bad effects could not be blamed on drug side-effects, for they occurred even among men who were never treated!).[12] What's even worse is that those with false-positive screening tests will experience only harm (regardless of the efficacy of early treatment). But even individuals with true-positive tests who receive efficacious treatment have had "healthy time" taken away from them; early diagnosis may not make folks live longer, but it surely makes all of them "sick" longer!

We've placed this discussion at the end of the chapter on diagnosis on purpose. In order to decide whether screening and case-finding do more good than harm, we'll have to consider the validity of claims about both the accuracy of the early diagnostic test and the efficacy of the therapy that follows it. We've summarized the guides for doing this in Table 5.9. Its elements are discussed in greater detail elsewhere.[13]

1. Is there RCT evidence that early diagnosis really leads to improved survival, or quality of life, or both?

Earlier detection will always appear to improve survival. The "lead time" between screen detection and usual detection (Figure 5.9) is always added to your apparent survival whether or not there is any real change. This is the first of several problems in evaluating early detection. Follow-up studies of placebo groups in RCTs have also taught us that patients who faithfully follow health advice (by volunteering

CARDS

Table 5.9 Guides for deciding whether a screening or early diagnostic maneuver does more good than harm

1. Is there RCT evidence that early diagnosis really leads to improved survival, or quality of life, or both?
2. Are the early diagnosed patients willing partners in the treatment strategy?
3. How do benefits and harms compare in different people and with different screening strategies?
4. Do the frequency and severity of the target disorder warrant the degree of effort and expenditure?

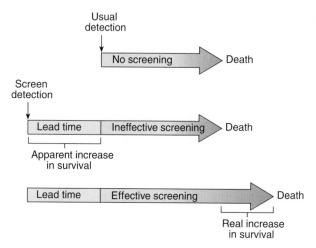

Figure 5.9 Lead-time. Time between screening and usual detection.

for screening or by taking their medicine) are different – and usually destined for better outcomes before they begin. Finally, early diagnostic maneuvers preferentially identify patients with slower progressing, more benign disease. As a result, the only evidence we can trust in determining whether early diagnosis does more good than harm is a true experiment in which individuals were randomly assigned.

As shown in Figure 5.10, this may be randomization to either (1) undergo the early detection test (and, if truly positive, treated for the target disorder) or to be left alone (and only treated if and when they developed symptomatic disease), or (2) be screened, and then positives randomized to early treatment or usual care. The latter sort of evidence has been used for showing the benefits (and harms) of detecting raised blood pressure and cholesterol. The former sort of evidence showed the benefit of mammography in women 50 years of age and older for reducing deaths from breast cancer,[††] and showed the uselessness (indeed, harm) of chest X-rays for lung cancer. Ideally,

---

[††]Because only about one-third of women whose breast cancers are diagnosed early go on to prolonged survival, even in this case the majority of positive screenees are harmed, not helped, by early detection.

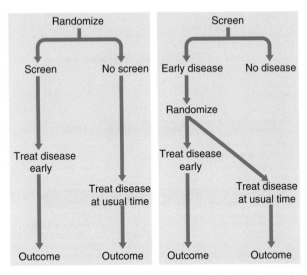

Figure 5.10 Two structures for randomized trials of the effectiveness of screening.

their follow-up will consider functional and quality-of-life outcomes as well as mortality and discrete clinical events, and we should not be satisfied when the only favorable changes are confined to "risk factors".

2. Are the early diagnosed patients willing partners in the treatment strategy?

Even when therapy is efficacious, patients who refuse or forget to take it cannot benefit from it and are left with only the damage produced by labeling. Early diagnosis will do more harm than good to these patients, and we forget the magnitude of this problem at their peril (even by self-report, only half of patients describe themselves as "compliant"). There are quick ways of diagnosing low compliance and we describe them to you in Chapter 4 (they comprise looking for non-attendance and non-responsiveness, and by non-confrontational questioning), but this is a diagnosis that you need to establish before, not after, you carry out any screening or case-finding.

3. How do benefits and harms compare in different people and with different screening strategies?

4. Do the frequency and severity of the target disorder warrant the degree of effort and expenditure?

These questions raise, at the levels of both our individual practice and our community, the unavoidable question of rationing. Is going after the early diagnosis of this condition worth sacrificing the other good we could accomplish by devoting our own or our town's resources to some other purpose?

We don't want to sound too gloomy here, and won't leave this topic without pointing you to places where you can find some of the triumphs of screening and case-finding: a good place to start is the Canadian Task Force on the Periodic Health Examination (which has recently been re-activated), where there are some rigorously evaluated ones.[14]

Tips for teaching around diagnostic tests

We usually begin by asking learners why we perform diagnostic tests, because they often respond: "To find out what's wrong with the patient (dummy!)" This provides an opening for helping them to recognize that diagnosis is not about finding absolute truth but about limiting uncertainty, and establishes both the necessity and the logical base for introducing probabilities, pragmatic test–treatment thresholds, and the like. It's also a time to get them to start thinking about what they're going to do with the results of the diagnostic test and about whether doing the test will really help their patient (maybe they'll conclude that the test isn't necessary!). A useful sequence is to elicit some disagreement between students, e.g., about a measurement or sign (but don't step in and suggest a "right" answer). The elicited disagreement can be used as an opening to unreliability and uncertainty. Comparison to a "gold standard" can introduce the issues of validity. While the formal calculations can be difficult, the qualitative ideas of SpIn and SnNout can be used, then be introduced to start students thinking about the accuracy and utility of a test.

When teaching about early diagnosis, we often challenge our learners with the statement: "Even when therapy is worthless, early diagnosis always improves survival!" and then help them recognize the distortions that arise from drawing conclusions about volunteers, from starting survival measurements unfairly early in screened patients, and from failing to recognize that early detection tests preferentially identify slowly – rather than rapidly – progressive disease. Once they've grasped those ideas, we think they're safe from the evangelists of early diagnosis.

References

1. Croskerry P. A universal model of diagnostic reasoning. *Acad Med.* 2009;84(8):1022–1028.

2. Moulton C, Regehr G, Mylopoulos M, MacRae MH. Slowing down when you should: A new model of expert judgment. *Acad Med.* 2007;82(suppl 10):S109–S116.

3. Heneghan C, Glasziou P, Thompson M, et al. Diagnostic strategies used in primary care. *BMJ.* 2009;338:b946.

4. Patterson C, Guyatt GH, Singer J, et al. Iron deficiency in the elderly: the diagnostic process. *Can Med Assoc J.* 1991;144(4):435–440.

5. Fleming KA. Evidence-based pathology. *Evid Based Med.* 1997;2:132.

6. Guyatt GH, Oxman AD, Ali M, et al. Laboratory diagnosis of iron deficiency anemia: an overview. *J Gen Intern Med.* 1992;7(2):145–153.

7. Richardson WS, Wilson M, McGinn T. Differential Diagnosis. In: Guyatt G, Rennie D, Meade M, Cook DJ, eds. *Users' guides to the medical literature. A manual for evidence-based clinical practice.* Chicago: AMA Press; 2008.

8. Bachmann LM, Kolb E, Koller MT, et al. Accuracy of Ottawa ankle rules to exclude fractures of the ankle and mid-foot: systematic review. *BMJ.* 2003;326(7386):417.

9. Whited JD, Grichnik JM. The rational clinical examination. Does this patient have a mole or a melanoma? *JAMA.* 1998;79(9):696–701.

10. Goodacre S, Sutton AJ, Sampson FC. Meta-analysis: the value of clinical assessment in the diagnosis of deep venous thrombosis. *Ann Intern Med.* 2005;143(2):129–139.

11. Shah KH, Metz HA, Edlow JA. Clinical prediction rules to stratify short-term risk of stroke among patients diagnosed in the emergency department with a transient ischemic attack. *Ann Emerg Med.* 2009;53(5):662–673.

12. Macdonald LA, Sackett DL, Haynes RB, et al. Labelling in hypertension: a review of the behavioural and psychological consequences. *J Chronic Dis.* 1984;37(12):933–942.

13. Barratt A, Irwig L, Glasziou P, et al. Users' guides to the medical literature: XVII. How to use guidelines and recommendations about screening. Evidence-Based Medicine Working Group. *JAMA*. 1999;281(21):2029–2034.

14. Canadian Task Force on the Periodic Health Examination. The periodic health examination. *Can Med Assn J*. 1979;121(9):1193–1254.

Further reading

Guyatt G, Rennie D, Meade M, Cook DJ, eds. *Users' guides to the medical literature. A manual for evidence-based clinical practice*. Chicago: AMA Press; 2008.

Haynes RB, Sackett DL, Guyatt GH, et al. *Clinical epidemiology: How to do clinical practice research*. Philadelphia: Lippincott Williams & Wilkins; 2006.

McGee S. *Evidence-based physical diagnosis*. 2nd ed. Philadelphia: Saunders; 2007.

McGinn T, Randolph A, Richardson S, et al. Clinical prediction guides. *Evid Based Med*. 1998;3:5–6.

5

6 Prognosis

Whether posed by our patients, colleagues or ourselves, we frequently need to consider questions about prognosis. For example, a patient newly diagnosed with Alzheimer dementia might ask, "What's going to happen to me?" Or a patient with a left-sided stroke might ask, "Will I regain function of my arm?" As clinicians, we might consider, "What is the prognosis in this patient with metastatic lung cancer?" "What is the risk of stroke in a patient with non-valvular atrial fibrillation?" Prognosis refers to determining the possible outcomes from a target disorder and the probability that they occur.

In order to answer these questions, and to make judgments about when to start and stop treatment, we need to evaluate evidence about prognosis for its validity, importance and relevance to our patients. The guides in Table 6.1 will help us tackle these issues. We'll consider the following clinical scenario to illustrate our discussion.

Clinical scenario

We see a 70-year-old man whom we recently diagnosed with dementia, most likely Alzheimer dementia. He comes to this appointment with his daughter who wants information on the progression of the disease and whether it will increase his risk of death. Her father had named her as his decision-maker for personal care and finances. His daughter wants to start planning for his future care as he has been living alone.

In response to this scenario, we posed the question, "In a 70-year-old man with newly diagnosed dementia, what is the risk of death?" Using *ACP Journal Club*, we searched the database using the term "dementia" and click on "prognosis" studies. We were quickly able to retrieve an article that might help us answer this question.[1] We also retrieved the original citation for this research article.[2]

Table 6.1 Is this evidence about prognosis valid?
1. Was a defined, representative sample of patients assembled at a common point in the course of their disease?
2. Was follow-up of study patients sufficiently long and complete?
3. Were objective outcome criteria applied in a "blind" fashion?
4. If subgroups with different prognoses are identified:
• Was there adjustment for important prognostic factors?
• Was there validation in an independent group of "test-set" patients?

Types of reports on prognosis

Several types of studies can provide information on the prognosis of a group of individuals with a defined problem or risk factor. The best evidence with which to answer our clinical question would come from a systematic review of prognosis studies. A systematic review that searches for and combines all relevant prognosis studies would be particularly useful for retrieving information about relevant patient subgroups. When assessing the validity of a systematic review, we'd need to consider the guides in Table 6.1 as well as those in Table 4.8. For example, in our search of *ACP Journal Club* described above, we retrieved a systematic review of the conversion rate to dementia in patients with mild cognitive impairment.[3] We can quickly see that a systematic search of the literature was completed for cohort studies that included patients with mild cognitive impairment (however, different definitions of mild cognitive impairment were used across studies). Outcomes were dementia or probable Alzheimer disease. However, at this time, relevant systematic reviews of prognosis studies are rare and we couldn't find one that addresses our clinical question. We'll focus the discussion in this chapter on individual studies.

Cohort studies (in which investigators follow one or more groups of individuals with the target disorder over time and monitor for occurrence of the outcome of interest) represent the best design for answering prognosis questions. Randomized trials can also serve as a source of prognostic information (particularly since they usually include detailed documentation of baseline data), although trial participants may not be entirely representative of the population with a disorder. The patients in the intervention arm can provide us with prognosis information for patients who receive treatment, whereas patients in the control arm can provide an estimate of prognosis for patients who don't receive the intervention. Case–control studies (in which investigators retrospectively determine prognostic factors by defining the exposures of cases who have already suffered the outcome of interest and controls that have not) are particularly useful when the outcome is rare or the required follow-up is long. However, the strength of inference that can be drawn from these studies is limited because of the potential for selection and measurement bias as discussed in Chapter 7.

Determining prognosis rarely relies on a single sign, symptom or laboratory test. Occasionally when completing our literature search we find articles describing tools that quantify the contributions that the clinical exam, laboratory and radiological investigations make in establishing a diagnosis or a prognosis for a patient. These tools that combine diagnostic and prognostic information are called clinical prediction guides and are more fully discussed in Chapter 5.

Are the results of this prognosis study valid?

1. Was a defined, representative sample of patients assembled at a common point in the course of their disease?

Ideally, the prognosis study we find would include the entire population of patients who ever lived who developed the disease, studied from the instant the disorder developed. Unfortunately, this is impossible and we'll have to determine how close the report we've found is to the ideal with respect to how the target disorder was defined and how participants were assembled. If the study sample fully reflects the spectrum of illness we find in our own practice, we are reassured. However, considering our clinical scenario, if the study that we found included only patients from a behavioural neurology unit that specialized in care for patients with dementia and agitation, we might not be satisfied that the sample is representative of the patients that we're interested in. These patients would have passed through a filter or referral process and thus don't reflect patients similar to our clinical scenario. The study should also describe the standardized criteria that were used to diagnose the target disorder.

But from what point in the disease should patients be followed? If investigators begin tracking outcomes only after some patients have already finished their course with the disease, then the outcomes for these patients might never be counted. Some would have recovered quickly, while others might have died quickly. So, to avoid missing outcomes by "starting the clock" too late, we look to see that study patients were included at a uniformly early time in the disease, ideally when it first becomes clinically manifest; this is called an "inception cohort".

6

A study that assembled patients at any defined, common point in their disease may provide useful information if we want information only about that stage of the disease. For example, we may want to understand the prognosis of patients with metastatic lung cancer. However, if observations were made at different points in the course of disease for various people in the cohort, the relative timing of outcome events would be difficult to interpret. For example, it would be difficult to interpret the results from a study designed to determine the prognosis of patients with rheumatoid arthritis that included patients with newly diagnosed disease as well as those who had the disease for 10 years or more. Similarly, it would be difficult to determine the prognosis of dementia in patients followed at a dementia clinic. These patients would likely be at different points in their illness. Ideally, we'd like to find a study in which participants are all at a similar stage in the course of the same disease.

Information about the study type and sampling method is usually found in the Abstract and Methods sections of the article. From the *ACP Journal Club* abstract we can quickly see that this study is an inception cohort including patients with dementia diagnosed by a geriatric mental state examination algorithm. Patients from a population cohort that included those from home and inpatient settings were interviewed every 2 years to diagnose dementia. Some patients may have been missed if they died rapidly after dementia onset because they were interviewed every 2 years. Those patients who were lost to follow-up or dropped out from the population cohort had higher mortality and these would have been missed from the inception cohort.

2. Was the follow-up of the study patients sufficiently long and complete?

Ideally, every patient in the cohort would be followed until they fully recover or develop one of the other disease outcomes. If follow-up is short, it may be that too few patients develop the outcome of interest and therefore we wouldn't have enough information to help us when advising our patients and in this case we'd better look for other evidence. For example, in our study of dementia, death at 1 month in patients newly diagnosed would not be helpful given the chronic, insidious nature of the disease. In contrast, if after years of follow-up, only a few adverse events have occurred, this good prognostic result is very useful in reassuring our patients about their future.

The more patients who are unavailable for follow-up, the less accurate the estimate of the risk of the outcome will be. The reasons for their loss are crucial. Some losses to follow-up are both unavoidable and mostly unrelated to prognosis (e.g., moving away to a different job) and these are not a cause for worry, especially if their numbers are small. But other losses might arise because patients die or are too ill to continue follow-up (or lose their independence and move in with family), and the failure to document and report their outcomes will reduce the validity of any conclusion the report draws about their prognosis.

Short of finding a report that kept track of every patient, how can we judge whether follow-up is "sufficiently complete"? There is no single answer for all studies, but we offer some suggestions to help. An analysis showing that the baseline demographics of these patients who were lost to follow-up are similar to those followed-up provides some reassurance that certain types of participants were not selectively lost, but such an analysis is limited by those characteristics that were measured at baseline. Investigators cannot control for unmeasured traits that may be important prognostically, and that may have been more or less prevalent in the lost participants than in the participants who were followed. We suggest considering the simple "5 and 20" rule: <5% loss probably leads to little bias; >20% loss seriously threatens validity; and in-between amounts cause intermediate amounts of trouble. While this may be easy to remember, it may oversimplify clinical situations in which the outcomes are infrequent. Alternatively, we could consider the "best" and "worst" case scenarios in an approach that we'll call a "sensitivity analysis". Imagine a study of prognosis wherein 100 patients enter the study, four die and 16 are lost to follow-up. A "crude" case-fatality rate would count the four deaths among the 84 with full follow-up, calculated as 4/84 = 4.8%. But what about the 16 who are lost? Some or all of them might have died too. In a "worst case" scenario, all would have died, giving a case-fatality rate of (4 known + 16 lost) = 20 out of (84 followed + 16 lost) = 100, or 20/100, i.e., 20% – four times the original rate that we calculated! *Note* that for the "worst case" scenario we've added the lost patients to both the numerator and the denominator of the outcome rate. On the other hand, in the "best case" scenario, none of the lost 16 would have died, yielding a case-fatality rate of 4 out of (84 followed + 16 lost), or 4/100, i.e. 4%. *Note* that for the "best case" scenario we've added the missing cases to just the denominator. While this "best case" of 4% may not differ much from the observed 4.8%, the "worst case" of 20% does differ meaningfully, and we'd probably

6

judge that this study's follow-up was not sufficiently complete and that it threatens the validity of the study. By using this simple sensitivity analysis, we can see what effect losses to follow-up might have on study results, which can help us judge whether the follow-up was sufficient to yield valid results. The larger the number of patients whose fate is unknown relative to the number who have the outcome, the more substantial the threat to validity.

> In the study that we found, all patients in the inception cohort were followed to the study completion.

3. Were objective outcome criteria applied in a blind fashion?

Diseases affect patients in many important ways; some are easy to spot and some are more subtle. In general, outcomes at both extremes – death or full recovery – are relatively easy to detect with validity, but assigning a cause of death is often subjective (as anyone who has completed a death certificate knows!). Review of death certificates often finds cardiac arrest recorded as the cause of death – but is the death due to pneumonia, pulmonary embolism, or something else? In between these extremes are a wide range of outcomes that can be more difficult to detect or confirm, and where investigators will have to use judgment in deciding how to count them (e.g., readiness for return to work, or the intensity of residual pain). To minimize the effects of bias in measuring these outcomes, investigators should have established specific criteria to define each important outcome and then used them throughout patient follow-up. We'd also want to satisfy ourselves that they are sufficiently objective for confirming the outcomes we're interested in. The occurrence of death is objective, but judging the underlying cause of death is prone to error (especially when it's based on death certificates) and can be biased unless objective criteria are applied to carefully gathered clinical information. But even with objective criteria, some bias might creep in if the investigators judging the outcomes also know about the patients' prior characteristics. Blinding is crucial if any judgment is required to assess the outcome, because unblinded investigators may search more aggressively for outcomes in people with the characteristic(s) felt to be of prognostic importance than in other individuals. In valid studies, investigators making judgments about clinical outcomes are kept "blind" to these patients' clinical characteristics and prognostic factors.

In the dementia study, the authors looked at death. Details of how death was determined need to be obtained from another study.[4] Participants were flagged on the Office of National Statistics NHS Central Register resulting in automatic notification of death. The need to track down this other paper highlights a challenge for the readers of clinical literature. With encouragement of authors to publish study protocols (often separately from the results), additional study details can be obtained. However, for the busy clinician this may mean reading two or three articles to find all of the relevant information that is needed for validity assessment. The *ACP Journal Club* abstract can provide some of these details but it doesn't provide details on how mortality was determined in the current study.

4. If subgroups with different prognoses are identified, was there adjustment for important prognostic factors and validation in an independent group of "test set" patients?

Prognostic factors are demographic (such as age, gender), disease specific (such as mitral valve prolapse with mitral regurgitation), or co-morbid (such as hypertension) variables that are associated with the outcome of interest. Prognostic factors need not be causal – and in fact they are often not – but they must be strongly associated with the development of an outcome to predict its occurrence. For example, although mild hyponatremia does not cause death, serum sodium is an important prognostic marker in congestive heart failure (individuals with congestive heart failure and hyponatremia have higher mortality rates than heart failure patients with normal serum sodium).[5]

Risk factors are often considered distinct from prognostic factors and include lifestyle behaviors and environmental exposures that are associated with the development of a target disorder. For example, smoking is an important risk factor for developing lung cancer but tumor stage is the most important prognostic factor in individuals who have lung cancer.

Often we will want to know whether subgroups of patients have different prognoses (e.g., among patients with mitral valve prolapse are those with moderate–severe mitral regurgitation or atrial fibrillation at increased risk of cardiovascular event or death compared with people without these findings). If a study reports that one group of patients had a different prognosis than another, first we need to see if there was any adjustment for known prognostic factors. By this we mean, did the authors make sure that these subgroup predictions are not being distorted by the unequal occurrence of another, powerful prognostic factor (such as would occur if patients with moderate–severe mitral regurgitation or atrial fibrillation were also more likely to have had a prior cardiac event than patients without these findings). There are both simple (e.g., stratified analyses displaying the prognoses of patients with mitral regurgitation separately for those with and without prior cardiac event) and fancy (e.g., multiple regression analyses that can take into account not only prior cardiac event but also left ventricular function) ways of adjusting for these other important prognostic factors. We can examine the Methods and Results sections to reassure ourselves that one of these methods has been applied, before we tentatively accept the conclusion about a different prognosis for the subgroup of interest. In our dementia study, presence of co-morbid disease could influence mortality. Similarly, co-morbid diseases could influence functional status. Are functional status and the presence of co-morbid diseases both factors that increase the risk of death in patients with dementia?

We say "tentatively" because the statistics of determining subgroup prognoses are about prediction, not explanation. They are indifferent to whether the prognostic factor is physiologically logical or a biologically nonsensical and random, non-causal quirk in the data (whether the patient lives on the north or the south side of the street or was born under a certain astrological sign). For this reason, the first time a prognostic factor is identified, there is no guarantee that it really does predict subgroups of patients with different prognoses – it could be the result of a chance difference in its distribution between patients with different prognoses. Indeed, if investigators were to search for multiple potential prognostic factors in the same dataset, a few would be likely to emerge on the basis of chance alone. The initial patient group in which prognostic factors are found is called a "training set" or "derivation set". Because of the risk of spurious, chance nomination of prognostic factors, we should look to see whether the predictive power of such factors has been confirmed in subsequent, independent groups of patients, termed "test sets" or "validation sets". To see if this was done, we'd look for a statement in the study's methods section, describing a pre-study intention to examine this specific group of prognostic factors, based on their appearance in a training set or previous study. If a second, independent study validates the predictive power of prognostic factors, we have a very useful "clinical prediction guide" (CPG) of the sort that we met earlier in this section and which were discussed fully in Chapter 4, but this time predicting our patient's outcome after he or she is diagnosed.

Blinding is also important when considering prognostic factors. If the person assessing the prognostic factor is aware that the patient had the outcome of interest, would they look harder for the potential prognostic factor?

> Multivariate analysis showed that functional impairment and older age were associated with higher risk for mortality and men had a higher risk for mortality than women. Investigators did not mention potential prognostic factors such as the presence of co-morbid conditions, different types of dementia or the effect of cognitive enhancers.

If the evidence about prognosis appears valid after considering the above guides, we can turn to examining its importance and applicability. But if we answered "no" to the questions above, we'd be better off searching for other evidence.

Is this valid evidence about prognosis important? (Table 6.2)

Table 6.2 Is this valid evidence about prognosis important?
1. How likely are the outcomes over time
2. How precise are the prognostic estimates?

CARDS

6

1. How likely are the outcomes over time?

Once we're satisfied that an article's conclusions are valid, we can examine it further to see how likely each outcome is over time. Typically, results from prognosis studies are reported in one of three ways: as a percentage of survival at a particular point in time (such as 1-year or 5-year survival rates); as median survival (the length of follow-up by which 50% of study patients have died); or as survival curves that depict, at each point in time, the proportion (expressed as a percentage) of the original study sample who have NOT yet had a specified outcome. In prognosis studies we often find results presented as Kaplan Meier curves, which are a type of survival curve.

Figure 6.1 shows four survival curves, each leading to a different conclusion. In panel A of Figure 6.1, virtually no patients had events by the end of the study, which could mean that either prognosis is very good for this target disorder (in which case the study is very useful to us), or the study is too short (in which case this study

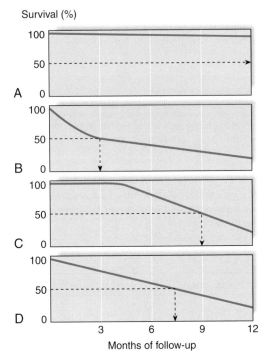

Figure 6.1 Prognosis shown as survival curves. (A) Good prognosis (or too short a study!). (B) Poor prognosis early, then slower increase in mortality, median survival of 3 months. (C) Good prognosis early, then worsening, with median survival of 9 months. (D) Steady prognosis.

isn't very helpful). In panels B, C and D, the proportion of patients surviving to 1 year (20%) is the same in all three graphs. And we could tell our patients that their chances of surviving for 1 year are 20%. However, the median survival (point at which half will have died) is very different – 3 months for B, versus 9 months for the disorder in Panel C. The survival pattern is a steady, uniform decline in Panel D and the median survival in this panel is approximately 7.5 months. These examples highlight the importance of considering median survival and survival curves in order to fully inform our patient about prognosis.

2. How precise are the prognostic estimates?

As we pointed out earlier, investigators study prognosis in a sample of diseased patients, not the whole population of everyone who has ever had the disease. Purely by the play of chance, then, a study repeated 100 times among different groups of patients (even with identical entry characteristics) is bound to generate different estimates of prognosis. In deciding whether a given set of prognostic results is important, we need some means of judging just how much the results could vary by chance alone. The confidence interval (CI) provides the range of values that are likely to include the true estimate and quantifies the uncertainty in measurement. By convention, the 95% CI is used and it represents the range of values within which we can be 95% sure that the population value lies. The narrower the CI, the more assured we can feel about the result. Note that if survival over time is the outcome of interest, earlier follow-up periods usually include results from more patients than later periods, so that survival curves are more precise (they provide narrower CIs) earlier in the follow-up. The text, tables or graphs of a good prognostic study include the CIs for its estimates of prognosis. If they don't, the calculators available on the book website can be used to do this calculation for you.

> From our study, we found that age, male sex (Hazard ratio 1.4) and functional impairment (2.1 [1.6–3.3]) were predictors of mortality. Education, social class and self-reported health didn't predict mortality. Median survival of male patients aged 70–79 was 4.6 years (3.0–8.6).

6

Can we apply this valid, important evidence about prognosis to our patient? (Table 6.3)

Table 6.3 Can we apply this valid, important evidence about prognosis to our patient?
1. Is our patient so different from those in the study that its results cannot apply?
2. Will this evidence make a clinically important impact on our conclusions about what to offer or tell our patient?

1. Is our patient so different from those in the study that its results cannot apply?

This guide asks us to compare our patients with those in the article, using descriptions of the study sample's demographic and clinical characteristics. Inevitably, some differences will turn up, so how similar is similar enough? We recommend framing the question the other way: are the study patients so different from ours that we should not use the results at all in making predictions for our patients? For most differences, the answer to this question is "no" and thus, we can use the study results to inform our prognostic conclusions.

2. Will this evidence make a clinically important impact on our conclusions about what to offer or tell our patient?

Evidence regarding a person's prognosis is clearly useful for deciding whether or not to initiate therapy, for monitoring therapy that has been initiated, and for deciding which diagnostic tests to order. If, for example, the study suggests an excellent prognosis for patients with a particular target disorder who didn't receive treatment, our discussions with patients would reflect these facts and would focus on whether any treatment should be started. If, on the other hand, the evidence suggests that the prognosis is poor without treatment (and if there are treatments that can make a meaningful difference), then our conversations with patients would reflect these facts and more likely lead us to treatment. Even when the prognostic evidence does not lead to a treat/don't treat decision, valid evidence can be useful in providing patients and families with the information they want about what the future is likely to hold for them and their illness.

> The patients in this study are similar to our patient. He has recently been diagnosed with Alzheimer disease. He also has a history of coronary artery disease which may increase his risk of death above those patients in the study. His functional status is currently good and he is able to do most of his activities of daily living. Based on the results of the study, we can provide an estimate of median survival to be approximately 5 years.

Practicing EBM in real-time

Sometimes we can't find the answers to our questions in high-quality, pre-appraised evidence resources and we must appraise the primary literature ourselves. After we've done this, it's useful to keep a copy of the appraisal in case the same question arises again. On the CD accompanying this book, we've provided the CATMaker software which you can use to make a record of your appraisal and then save it in your own database. We've found this software to be a useful teaching tool but we don't use it routinely in clinical practice because it takes too long. Instead we developed an abbreviated version that allows us to quickly record our question, the main study details, the results and any comments/ concerns about the study. We can save this as a 'word' file for our PC or for our PDA. Using this tool, we can develop our own database of topics that we encounter in our own practice. We've provided this CQ log on the accompanying CD and you can download it to your PDA – you can use it to log your clinical questions and the answers to those you've managed to track down. But keep in mind that these should have an expiry date on them! If we have colleagues close by, we can share the work and collaborate on these.

References

1. Molloy DW. Age, sex and functional impairment predicted risk for mortality in incident dementia at 14 year follow-up. *ACP J Club.* 2008;149(1):13.

2. Xie J, Brayne C, Matthews FE, the MRC Cognitive Function and Ageing Study Collaborators. Survival times in people with dementia: analysis from population based cohort study with 14 year follow-up. *BMJ.* 2008;336(7638):258–262.

3. Burke D, ACP Journal Club. Review: long-term annual conversion rate to dementia was 3.3% in older adults with mild cognitive impairment. *Ann Intern Med.* 2009;150(8):JC4–JC13.

4. Neale R, Brayne C, Johnson AL. Cognition and survival: an exploration in a large multicentre study of the population aged 65 years and over. *Int J Epidemiol.* 2001;30(6):1383–1388.

5. Mettauer B, Rouleau JL, Bichet D, et al. Sodium and water excretion abnormalities in congestive heart failure: determinant factors and clinical implications. *Ann Intern Med.* 1986;105(2):161–167.

6

Further reading

Haynes RB, Sackett DL, Guyatt G, et al. *Clinical epidemiology: How to do clinical practice research.* Philadelphia: Lippincott Williams & Wilkins; 2006.

Guyatt G, Rennie D, Meade M, et al., eds. *Users' guides to the medical literature. A manual for evidence-based clinical practice.* Chicago: AMA press; 2008.

7 Harm

The media constantly bombards us with concerns about potentially harmful interventions, leading to questions by us and our patients such as, "Does living close to hydroelectric power lines increase the risk of cancer?", "Do statins cause cancer?", "Does the MMR vaccine cause autism?" "Do NSAIDs increase the risk of cardiovascular mortality?" In Chapter 2, our patient was unaware of the harmful effects of beta-carotene and vitamin E supplementation and, in Chapter 4, our patient's daughter wondered about the potential harms and benefits from antipsychotic medications. Along with our patients, we often need to make judgments about whether these medical interventions and environmental agents could be harmful.

To make these judgments, we need to be able to evaluate evidence about causation for its validity, importance and direct relevance to our patients. Assessing the validity of the evidence is crucial if we are to avoid drawing the false-positive conclusion that an agent does cause an adverse event when, in truth, it does not; or the false-negative conclusion that an agent does not cause an adverse event when, in truth, it does. Clinical disagreements about whether a patient has had an adverse drug reaction are not uncommon – and just because an adverse event occurred during treatment, it does not inevitably follow that the adverse event occurred because of that treatment.

The guides in Table 7.1 can help us to appraise the validity of an article about a putative harmful agent. We'll consider the following clinical scenario to illustrate our discussion.

7

Clinical scenario

During a routine health maintenance visit, we see a 45-year-old woman who complains of urge incontinence which has become progressively worse over the last 2 years, significantly impacting on her quality of life. Her past history is remarkable for three pregnancies (she had urge incontinence associated with each of these) and forceps were used during two of the births. She takes lorazepam occasionally at night for difficulty sleeping. She is on no other medications and has no smoking history. Her caffeine intake consists of 750 ml (25 oz) of coffee per day. Her clinical examination is unremarkable except for visible urine leakage when she is asked to cough while in the lithotomy position. Her post-void residual urine volume is 20 ml and a urinalysis is unremarkable. She recently read in an online chat group of women with urinary incontinence that caffeine can cause urinary incontinence and wants to know if this is true or if there are other factors that could be contributing to her problem.

CARDS

Table 7.1 Is this evidence about harm valid?

1. Were there clearly defined groups of patients, similar in all important ways other than exposure to the treatment or other cause?
2. Were treatments/exposures and clinical outcomes measured in the same ways in both groups? (Was the assessment of outcomes either objective or blinded to exposure?)
3. Was the follow-up of the study patients sufficiently long (for the outcome to occur in a large enough number of patients) and complete (so that no or very few patients were lost to follow-up)?
4. Do the results of the harm study fulfill some of the diagnostic tests for causation?
   - Is it clear that the exposure preceded the onset of the outcome?
   - Is there a dose–response gradient?
   - Is there any positive evidence from a "dechallenge–rechallenge" study?
   - Is the association consistent from study to study?
   - Does the association make biological sense?

In response to this scenario, we posed the question, "In a woman with urge incontinence, does caffeine consumption cause urinary incontinence?" Using the Clinical Queries function of PubMed (with the search terms "urinary incontinence" and "caffeine") we were able to identify an article that might help us to answer this question.[1]

Types of reports on harm/etiology

As we discovered in Chapter 4, ideally the best evidence that we can find about the effects of therapy (and putative harmful agents) comes from systematic reviews. Individual randomized trials are seldom large enough to detect rare adverse events with precision – emphasizing the need to search for a systematic review. A systematic review that combines all relevant randomized trials or cohort studies might provide us with sufficiently large numbers of patients to detect even rare adverse events. When assessing the validity of such a systematic review, we need to consider the guides in Table 7.1 as well as those in Table 4.8. For example, at journal club recently, we were interested in whether statins were safe in patients with liver disease. We found a systematic review published in 2008[2] that searched Medline and abstracts of medical meetings to attempt to answer this question. Very few articles were identified. For patients with elevated liver enzymes (defined as >1 × the upper limit of normal), a pooled subgroup analysis of three randomized trials and information from two retrospective cohort studies found no significant increased risk of elevation in liver enzymes of three times the upper limit of normal or higher. Overall, the limited evidence available suggests that statins are safe, even in patients with cirrhosis. However, this article highlights a challenge for us as users of the literature, which we also mentioned in Chapter 4. Systematic reviews can only synthesize the literature that is available. Studies have shown that most trials are small and don't have sufficient sample size or follow-up duration to provide precise estimates of risks of adverse events.[3] Finally, unfortunately reviews of harm/etiology aren't common and the discussion in this chapter will focus on randomized trials, cohort, case-control studies and cross-sectional studies.

Are the results of this harm/etiology study valid?

1. Were there clearly defined groups of patients, similar in all important ways other than exposure to the treatment or other cause?

Ideally our search would yield a systematic review or a randomized trial in which women had been allocated, by a system analogous to tossing a coin, to caffeine (amount of caffeine could be specified) consumption (the top row in Table 7.2, whose total is a + b), or some comparison intervention (decaffeinated beverages) or placebo (the bottom row in Table 7.2, whose total is c + d) and then followed over time for the development of urinary incontinence. Randomization would tend to make the two treatment groups identical for all other causes of urinary incontinence (and we'd look for baseline differences in other putative causal agents between the groups), so we'd likely consider any statistically significant increase in

CARDS

Table 7.2 Studies of whether caffeine consumption causes urinary incontinence

	Adverse outcome		Totals
	Present (Case)	**Absent (Controls)**	
Exposed to treatment (RCT or cohort)	a	b	a+b
Not exposed to treatment (RCT or cohort)	c	d	c+d
Totals	a+c	b+d	a+b+c+d

urge incontinence (adjusted for any important baseline differences) in the intervention group to be valid. Randomized control trials, however, are ill-suited (in size, duration, and ethics) for evaluating most harmful exposures, and we often have to make do with evidence from other types of studies.* Consider how tough it would be to complete a study in which we randomize women to caffeine consumption vs no caffeine consumption – and returning to the questions posed at the beginning of this chapter, it would be impossible to randomize families to live in a house either close to or at a distance from power lines to determine the impact on cancer development! Unfortunately, the validity of the study designs used to detect harm is inversely proportional to their feasibility.

In the first of these alternatives, a cohort study, a group of participants who are exposed (a+b) to the treatment (or putative harmful agent) and a group or participants who aren't exposed (c+d) to it are followed for the development of the outcome of interest (a or c). Returning to our example, a cohort study would include a group of women with a history of caffeine consumption and a group without and then the risk of urge incontinence would be determined in each. As we discussed in Chapter 4, in observational studies such as cohort studies, the decision to prescribe and accept exposure is based on the patient's and/or physician's preferences and it is not randomized. As a result, "exposed" patients may differ from "non-exposed" patients in important determinants of

---

*There are many examples where we've been misled by observational studies whose results were found to be proved wrong when these ideas were tested in randomized trials. Consider the data from observational studies which showed the benefits of HRT in women, particularly a decreased risk of cardiovascular mortality. It was only when the Women's' Health Initiative was completed that we had cause for concern that indeed we were increasing risk of cardiovascular mortality with HRT!

the outcome (such determinants are called confounders).[†] For example, consider a paper that looks at the relationship between estrogen use and the risk of urinary incontinence. Increasing age is associated with urinary incontinence and older women may be more likely to use estrogen. Therefore age could be a confounder when comparing the risk of urinary incontinence in women using and not using estrogen. Investigators must document the characteristics of both cohorts of patients and either demonstrate their comparability or adjust for the confounders they identify (using for example, special statistical techniques like multivariable analysis). Of course, adjustments can only be made for confounders that are already known and have been measured, so we have to be careful when interpreting cohort studies.[‡]

Cohort studies can be prospective or retrospective. In retrospective studies, we already have the data on outcomes that have occurred and we look before these have happened to select exposed and unexposed individuals. In prospective studies, we identify our exposed and non-exposed participants and follow them for the development of the outcome. We can easily see which study type is easier (and cheaper!) to perform. Studies using administrative databases (such as claims' databases) are examples of the former but there are some limitations to these databases that we need to consider when we're reading research studies that have used these resources. First, they were not developed for research use and thus often don't contain all the information that would be useful including data on severity of illness.[4] Second, coding is often inaccurate and also incomplete because there may be limited space for secondary diagnoses in these databases.[5] Third, we can only find events for which there are codes.[5] Fourth, the databases may not include the entire population. For example, the Medicare files in the USA include only those patients eligible to receive Medicare, which includes people ≥ 65 and, some people under ≥ 65 with disabilities and all people with end-stage renal disease requiring renal replacement therapy.

Professors Doll and Hill[6] highlighted the importance of completing prospective cohort studies in 1950 when they were looking at the possible association between smoking and lung cancer. Several retrospective studies found an association between smoking and lung cancer but the size of the association varied across the studies. There was much

7

[†]Confounders have the three properties of being: extraneous to the question posed; determinants of the outcome; and unequally distributed between exposed and non-exposed participants.
[‡]As we mentioned in Chapter 4, this is another great thing about randomization – it balances the groups for confounders that we haven't identified yet!

discussion around the association but it was not extended to causation and they determined that this debate would not be advanced by yet another retrospective study. Instead, they advocated a prospective approach, whereby the development of the disease could be determined over time in people whose smoking habits were already known. This led to their landmark study published in 1951 showing the mortality of male physicians in relation to their smoking habits.[6] Remarkably, Professor Doll and colleagues continued this work for more than 50 years and published an update to the paper in 2004.[7]

If the outcome of interest is rare or takes a long time to develop (e.g., the development of cancer or asbestosis), even large cohort studies may not be feasible and we will have to look for alternatives, such as case–control studies. In this study design, people with the outcome of interest (a + c) are identified as "cases" and those without it (b + d) are selected as controls and the proportion of each group who were exposed to the putative agent (a/a + c or b/b + d) is assessed retrospectively. There is even more potential for confounding with case–control studies than with cohort studies because confounders that are transient or lead to early death can't be measured. For example, if patients are selected from hospital sources, the relationship between outcome and exposure will be distorted if patients who are exposed are more likely to be admitted to the hospital than are the unexposed. This was illustrated nicely in a systematic review that looked at the association between vasectomy and prostate cancer – the relative risk of prostate cancer following vasectomy was significantly elevated in hospital-based studies (1.98 [95% CI 1.37–2.86]) but not in population-based ones (1.12 [95% CI 0.96–1.32]).[8]

Inappropriate selection of control participants can lead to false associations and "control" participants should have the same opportunity for exposure to the putative agent as the "case" participants. For example, if we found a case–control study evaluating the association between benzodiazepines and urinary incontinence that assembled women with urinary incontinence as cases but excluded patients with a history of falls or anxiety disorder from the control group (who might be at increased risk of exposure to benzodiazepines), we'd be right to wonder whether an observed association was spurious.

We can see that this study design easily lends itself to the exploration of possible relationships between many exposures and the outcome of interest (especially with the common usage and availability of administrative databases). Therefore we must bear in mind that if a large number of potential associations were explored, a statistically significant finding could be based on chance alone.

When we're searching for an answer to an etiology question, the articles that we find most commonly (because they're cheaper and easier to do!) describe cross-sectional studies and unfortunately, these studies are susceptible to even more bias than case–control studies. In a cross-sectional study, the authors would look at a group of women with urge incontinence (a + c) and a group without (b + d) and assess caffeine consumption (a or b) in both. Exposure and outcomes are measured at the same time – and this highlights one of the major problems with this study type; which came first? Also, as with cohort and case–control studies, adjustment must be made for confounders. These studies may be helpful for hypothesis generation.

Finally, we may only find case reports of one patient (or a case series of a few patients) who developed an adverse event while receiving the suspected exposure (cell a). If the outcome is unusual and dramatic enough (phocomelia in children born to women who took thalidomide), such case reports and case series may be enough to answer our question. But because these studies lack comparison groups, they are usually only sufficient for hypothesis generation and thus highlight the need for other studies.

We usually find information about the study type and how participants were selected in the Abstract and Methods sections of the article. Information describing participants is often found in the Results section.

To answer Question 1 in Table 7.1, we read the article we found which describes a case–control study that established a group of women with detrusor instability and a group without, and assessed caffeine consumption in both groups. Detrusor instability was diagnosed if the women had symptoms of urge incontinence and had evidence of bladder contraction and leakage on urodynamic testing. Control participants had stress incontinence and ideally we'd want the control group to include age-matched continent women. Overall, we're happy that the patients in the case and control groups were similar.

7

2. Were treatments/exposures and clinical outcomes measured in the same ways in both groups? (Was the assessment of outcomes either objective or blinded to exposure?)

We should place greater confidence in studies in which treatment exposures and clinical outcomes were measured in the same way in both groups. Moreover, we would prefer that the outcomes assessors were blind to the exposure in cohort studies and to the outcome and study hypothesis in case–control studies. Consider a report describing a cohort study looking at the association between coffee consumption and urinary incontinence. We'd be concerned if the investigator searched more aggressively for urinary incontinence in women who were known to have heavy caffeine consumption. Indeed, when the outcomes assessors aren't blinded to the exposure, they may search harder for the disease in the exposed group and identify disease that might otherwise have been unnoticed. Now consider a case–control study evaluating the same potential association – if the investigator is not blind to the outcome or study hypothesis, they might look harder for a history of heavy caffeine consumption in women whom they know to have urinary incontinence. Similarly, women with urinary incontinence might have considered their situation more carefully and may have greater ability or incentive to recall possible exposure. Thus, we'd feel more assured about the study if the report described that the patients (and their interviewers) were blinded to the study hypothesis.

This discussion raises another, finer point regarding the source of the information about the outcome or exposure of interest. Sometimes in articles, we find that the investigators use health records to seek information about the exposure or outcome retrospectively and as clinicians who complete these records (and often have to use them at a later date to dictate a discharge summary), we have to ask ourselves if we consider this method sufficiently accurate. Consider for example, the impact on a study's results if the likelihood of the data being recorded differs between the groups. Similarly, information from some administrative databases might not be as accurate as that collected prospectively (although for certain types of information such as drug usage, a drug claims database will provide more accurate information than patient or physician recall).

Information about measurement of the exposure or outcome is usually included in the Methods and Results sections. In the study that we found, participants in both the control and the case groups were asked to complete a 48 hour voiding diary before urodynamic testing consisting of a structured intake and output record of the type and amount of fluid. They were asked to record their intake of coffee, tea, cola and cocoa using a measuring cup. The reproducibility of this diary was assessed in a random sample of women after an interval of 1 week. It does not state if the patients were aware of the study hypothesis. Health records were reviewed to obtain information about potential confounders including parity and smoking history.

3. Was the follow-up of the study patients sufficiently long (for the outcome to occur) and complete?

Ideally, we'd like to see that no patients were lost to follow-up because lost patients may have had outcomes that would affect the conclusions of the study. For example, in a cohort study looking at the association between urinary incontinence and caffeine consumption, imagine the impact on its results if a large number of women in the caffeine cohort left the study – we wouldn't know if it was because they developed urge incontinence and left the study to seek treatment, or because they became frustrated with the study. As mentioned in Chapter 4, evidence-based journals of secondary publication like *ACP Journal Club* use a 20% loss to follow-up as an exclusion criterion because it would be rare for a study to suffer such a loss and not have its results affected. And, we'd like to see that the patients were followed for an appropriate period of time. For example, if we found a study of the association between cancer and living close to hydroelectric wires that followed patients for only a few weeks, we wouldn't be able to distinguish a true- from a false-negative association.

4. Do the results of the harm study satisfy some of the diagnostic tests for causation?

Investigators may identify an association between an exposure and outcome but is the exposure causative? "Diagnostic tests for causation" can help us with this concern including the following:

- *Is it clear that the exposure preceded the onset of the outcome?* We'd want to make sure that the exposure (e.g., caffeine) occurred prior to the development of the adverse outcome (e.g., urinary incontinence). When Professors Doll and Hill[6] were doing their work on smoking and lung cancer, this was a key issue they identified in their rationale for the prospective study – did the smoking exposure happen before the development of lung cancer?

- *Is there a dose–response gradient?* The demonstration of an increasing risk (or severity) of the adverse event with increasing exposure (increased dose and/or duration) to the putative causal agent strengthens the association. For example, heavy smokers are at greater risk of cancer than occasional/light smokers.[9] In the case–control study that we found looking at caffeine consumption and urinary incontinence, people with greater caffeine consumption (>400 mg/day) had a higher risk of urinary incontinence than those with lower caffeine consumption.

7

- *Is there any positive evidence from a "dechallenge–rechallenge" study?* We'd like to see that the adverse outcome decreases or disappears when the treatment is withdrawn and worsens or reappears when it is reintroduced. Returning to our clinical scenario, it would be useful to know if caffeine consumption is reduced or stopped, does the urinary incontinence improve in the heavy caffeine users? This information is not available from the study. In the 2004 study on tobacco use and mortality, Professor Doll and colleagues were able to show that smoking cessation leads to a survival benefit. Stopping smoking at age 60, 50, 40 or 30 gains approximately 3, 6, 9 or 10 years, respectively.[7]

- *Is the association consistent from study to study?* If we were able to find multiple studies or, better yet, a systematic review of the question, we could determine whether the association between exposure and the adverse event is consistent from study to study. While there aren't other studies looking at the association between caffeine use and urinary incontinence, we found a small trial evaluating caffeine reduction which decreased urinary symptoms in women with incontinence.[10] Two other studies found similar results when caffeine reduction was part of a multicomponent intervention for women with urinary incontinence.

Does the association make biological sense? If the association between exposure and outcome makes biological sense (in terms of pathophysiology, etc.), a causal interpretation becomes more plausible. The authors of our study theorize that caffeine has an excitatory effect on detrusor smooth muscle possibly through the release of intracellular calcium. (Keep in mind that this theory is based on data from animal models!)

Are the valid results of this harm study important?

If the study we find fails to satisfy the first three minimum standards in Table 7.1, we'd probably be better off abandoning it and continuing our search. But if we are satisfied that it meets these minimum guides, we need to decide if the association between exposure and outcome is sufficiently strong and convincing for us to do something about it. By this, we mean looking at the risk or odds of the adverse effect with (as opposed to without) exposure to the treatment; the higher the risk or odds, the stronger the association and the more we should be impressed by it. We can use the guides in Table 7.3 to determine if the valid results of the study are important.

CARDS

Table 7.3 Are the valid results of this harm study important?

1. What is the magnitude of the association between the exposure and outcome?
2. What is the precision of the estimate of the association between the exposure and the outcome?

1. What is the magnitude of the association between the exposure and outcome?

As noted above, questions of etiology can be answered by several different study designs. Different study designs require different methods for estimating the strength of association between exposure to the putative cause and the outcome of interest. In randomized trials and cohort studies, this association is often described by calculating the risk (or incidence) of the adverse event in the exposed (or treated) patients relative to that in the unexposed (or untreated) patients. This relative risk is calculated as: $[a/(a+b)]/[c/(c+d)]$ (from Table 7.2). For example, if 1000 patients receive a treatment and 20 of them develop the outcome of interest:

$a = 20$ and $a/(a+b) = 2\%$

(The risk of experiencing the outcome with treatment is 2%)

If 1000 patients didn't receive the treatment and 2 experienced the outcome:

$c = 2$ and $c/(c+d) = 0.2\%$

(The risk of experiencing the outcome in the absence of treatment is 0.2%)

Therefore the relative risk (RR) becomes:

$2\%/0.2\% = 10$

This means that patients receiving the treatment are 10 times as likely to experience the outcome as patients not receiving the treatment.

From the preceding example, we can see that to calculate the RR we needed a group of treated participants and a group who didn't receive

7

treatment and then we determined the proportion with the outcome in each group. But, in case–control studies we can't calculate the RR because the investigator selects the people with the outcomes (rather than those with the exposure) and therefore we can't calculate the "incidence". Instead we look to an indirect estimate of the strength of association in a case–control study and this is called an odds ratio (or relative odds). Referring to Table 7.2 it is calculated as "ad/bc". The odds of experiencing the outcome in exposed patients is a/b. The odds of experiencing the outcome in those not exposed is c/d. We can then compare the odds of experiencing the outcome in those who are exposed with the odds of experiencing the outcome in those who are not exposed: (a/b)/(c/d) or ad/bc.

If for example, 100 cases of patients with urge incontinence are identified and it's found that 90 of them had a history of caffeine consumption, a = 90 and c = 10. If 100 patients without the outcome are assembled and it is found that 45 of them received the exposure, b = 45 and d = 55, the odds ratio (OR) becomes:

$$(90/45)/(10/55)$$
$$= 90 \times 55/45 \times 10$$
$$= 11$$

This means that the odds of experiencing the adverse event for people who had a history of caffeine consumption was 11 times that of those who didn't have the same exposure.

Note that risks = odds/(1 + odds) and odds = (risk/1 – risk). We did this same calculation in Chapter 5 when we were converting pre-test probabilities to pre-test odds to allow us to multiply this by the likelihood ratio. We then used the second equation to convert from post-test odds to post-test probability.

ORs and RRs >1 indicate that there is an increased risk of the adverse outcome associated with the exposure. And when the RR or OR = 1, the adverse event is no more likely to occur with than without the exposure to the suspected agent.[§] (Conversely, when the ORs and RRs <1, the adverse event is less likely to occur with the exposure to the putative agent than without.) It should also be noted that when event rates are very low, the RR and OR approximate each other. And, they are close when the treatment effect is small. This is

---

[§]Remember that a ratio is just a numerator and a denominator. When the numerator is the same as the denominator, the ratio is 1, i.e., there is no difference between the numerator and denominator (or between the risk or odds of events).

sometimes a cause for confusion because often in articles we find ORs have been calculated but the authors report and discuss them as RRs. **

How big should the RR or OR be for us to be impressed? This brings us back to issues of validity because we have to consider the strength of the study design when we're evaluating the strength of the association. As we discussed earlier in this chapter, a well-done randomized trial is susceptible to less bias than either a cohort or case–control study. Therefore we'd be satisfied with a smaller increase in risk from a randomized trial than from a cohort or case–control study. Because cohort and even more so, case–control studies are susceptible to many biases, we want to ensure that the OR is greater than that which would result from bias alone. As rules of thumb (and taking into account the features of the individual study/ies), we might not want to label an odds ratio from a case–control study as impressive unless it is >4 for minor adverse events and we'd set this value at progressively lower levels as the severity of the adverse event increases. There is less potential bias in cohort studies and therefore we might regard a relative risk of >3 as convincing for more severe adverse events.

Professor Les Irwig (personal communication) has provided another useful tip when looking at the strength of the association. It requires us to find a report that includes some adjustment for potential confounders. He suggests that we compare the unadjusted measure of association with one in which at least one known confounder has been adjusted out. If this adjustment produces a large decline in the RR or OR, we should be suspicious of a spurious association. If in contrast, the adjusted OR or RR is stable with this adjustment, or if it rises rather than falls, our confidence in the validity of the association would be greater.

7

In our study, high caffeine intake was associated with detrusor instability but this OR declined slightly after adjusting for smoking history and age (OR 2.7 vs 2.4 after adjustment), which decreases our confidence in the validity of the association slightly.

**Note that risks = odds/(1 + odds) and odds = risk/(1 − risk). We used the second equation in Chapter 5 when we were converting pre-test probabilities to pre-test odds to allow us to multiply this by the likelihood ratio. We then used the first equation to convert from post-test odds to post-test probability.

Although the OR and RR tell us about the strength of the association, we need to translate this into some measure that is useful and intelligible both to us and our patient. This is of particular importance when the discussion concerns a medication or some other medical intervention we and our patient are considering. For this, we can turn to the number needed to harm (NNH), which tells us the "number of patients who need to be exposed to the putative causal agent to produce one additional harmful event". The NNH can be calculated directly from trials and cohort studies in a fashion analogous to the NNT, but this time as the reciprocal of the difference in adverse event rates:

$$= 1 / [a / (a + b)] - [c / (c + d)].$$

For an OR derived from a case–control study, the calculation is more complex (remember, we can't determine "incidence" directly in a case–control study). Its scary formula reads (if the OR <1): (and don't worry, we won't test you on this!)

$$1 - [PEER(1 - OR)] / PEER(1 - PEER)(1 - OR)$$

and if the OR >1:

$$1 + [PEER \times (OR - 1)] / PEER(1 - PEER)(OR - 1)$$

where PEER is the patient expected event rate (the adverse event rate among individuals who are not exposed to the putative cause). We've made this easier for you by providing some typical PEERs and ORs and summarizing them in Tables 7.4 and 7.5. As you can see, for different PEERs, the same OR can lead to very different NNHs and it is therefore important that we do our best to estimate our patient's expected event rate when calculating the NNH. For example, if the OR is 0.90 and the PEER was 0.005, the NNH would be 2000, but if the PEER was 0.40 (and the OR is 0.90), the NNH would be 40. We'll consider individual patients in further detail later.

Practicing and teaching EBM in real-time 1

The above formula is complex and we rarely use it. If the answer we're looking for isn't in Table 7.4 and 7.5, we use the EBM calculator to quickly convert an OR to an NNH. Firing up the EBM calculator on the website (www.cebm.utoronto.ca/practice/ca/statscal/orToNnt.htm) or from the accompanying CD, we can insert our OR of 0.90 and our PEER of 0.005 and at the click of a button, the NNH is calculated. We can also download this calculator to our PDA for quick usage (Fig. 7.1).

Table 7.4 Translating odds ratios (ORs) to NNHs when ORs <1

Patient expected event rate (PEER)	For ORs LESS than 1						
	0.9	0.9	0.7	0.6	0.5	0.4	0.3
0.05	209[a]	104	69	52	41	34	29[b]
0.10	110	54	36	27	21	18	15
0.20	61	30	20	14	11	10	8
0.30	46	22	14	10	8	7	5
0.40	40	19	12	9	7	6	4
0.50	38	18	11	8	6	5	4
0.70	44	20	13	9	6	5	4
0.90	101[c]	46	27	18	12	9	4[d]

[a]The relative risk reduction (RRR) here is 10%.
[b]The RRR here is 49%.
[c]The RRR here is 1%.
[d]The RRR here is 9%.
Adapted from John Geddes (pers comm 1999).

Table 7.5 Translating odds ratios (ORs) to NNHs when ORs >1

Patient expected event rate (PEER)	For odds ratios GREATER than 1						
	1.1	1.25	1.5	1.75	2	2.25	2.5
0.05	212	86	44	30	23	18	16
0.10	113	46	24	16	13	10	9
0.20	64	27	14	10	8	7	6
0.30	50	21	11	8	7	6	5
0.40	44	19	10	8	6	5	5
0.50	42	18	10	8	6	6	5
0.70	51	23	13	10	9	8	7
0.90	121	55	33	25	22	19	18

The numbers in the body of the table are the "number needed to harm" (NNHs) for the corresponding ORs at that particular PEER.
Adapted from John Geddes (pers comm 1999).

We find it much easier to use NNTs/NNHs when we're teaching. Many of the housestaff we work with carry iPhones or Blackberries and we also find that with so many PCs available on the wards and in clinics, we can easily use this web version of the calculator. It's also an opportunity for teaching around how we would communicate this information about

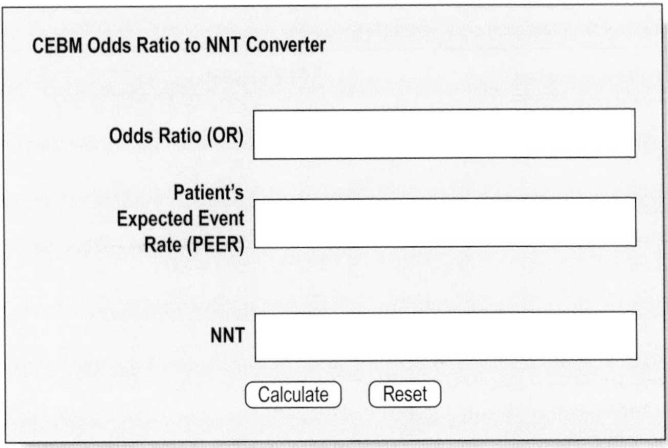

CEBM Odds Ratio to NNT Converter

Odds Ratio (OR)

Patient's
Expected Event
Rate (PEER)

NNT

(Calculate) (Reset)

Figure 7.1 Using the EBM calculator to convert OR to NNH. Note that, because we are increasing the risk of a bad event, we calculate an NNH, not an NNT. This version of the calculator doesn't recognize the difference between NNT and NNH.

risk for our patient or to a colleague. We've found it fun to give each trainee 1 minute to explain the results/bottom line to a colleague. Other members of the team then give feedback to the trainee.

1. What is the precision of the estimate of the association between the exposure and outcome?

In addition to looking at the magnitude of the RR or OR, we need to look at its precision by examining the confidence interval (CI) around it. Credibility is highest when the entire CI is narrow and remains within a clinically importantly increased risk. For example, we found a systematic review that described a significant association between serum homocysteine level and risk of ischemic heart disease.[11] From this study, the adjusted OR for ischemic heart disease or stroke associated with a 25% lower serum homocysteine level was 0.89 with 95% CI 0.83–0.96. The upper limit of this CI is the smallest estimate of the strength of the association and this approximates 1! Similarly if a study finds no association, the limits of the CI could tell us if a potentially important positive result (indicating an association) has been excluded. In our

> **Table 7.6** Guides for deciding whether valid important evidence about harm can be applied to our patient
>
> 1. Is our patient so different from those included in the study that its results cannot apply?
> 2. What are our patient's risks of benefit and harm from the agent?
> 3. What are our patient's preferences, concerns and expectations from this treatment?
> 4. What alternative treatments are available?

caffeine study, the OR was 2.4 (adjusted for age and smoking) with 95% CI 1.1–6.5. Note that the lower limit of the CI is close to 1 and as you will recall, when the OR approximates 1, the adverse event is no more likely to occur with than without the exposure to the suspected agent.

Once we have decided that the evidence we have found is both valid and important, we need to consider if it can be applied to our patient (Table 7.6).

Can this valid and important evidence about harm be applied to our patient?

1. Is our patient so different from those included in the study that its results cannot apply?

As emphasized in previous chapters, the issue is not whether our patient fulfils all the inclusion criteria for the study we found, but whether our patient is so different from those in the study that its results are of no help to us. See Chapter 4 for further discussion of this issue.

2. What are our patient's risks of benefit and harm from the agent?

We need to consider both the potential benefits and harms from the agent. For each patient, we need to individualize these risks. To apply the results of a study to an individual patient, we need to estimate our patient's risk of the adverse event if she were not exposed to the putative cause. There's a hard way and an easy way to tackle this. The hard way requires searching for good evidence on prognosis, and the much easier way requires estimating the risk relative to that of unexposed individuals in the study. Just as with NNTs in Chapter 4, we can express this as a decimal fraction (called "f"): if our patient is at half the risk of study patients, $f = 0.5$; if our patient is at three times the risk, $f = 3$. The study NNH can then be divided by f to produce the NNH for our individual patient. For example, suppose a study found we'd only need to treat 150 people with a statin to cause one additional person to experience myalgias. But if we think our patient is at twice the risk of the study patients, f = 2 and 150/2 generates an NNH of 75. If, on the other hand, we thought our patient was at one-third the risk (f = 0.33), the NNH for patients like ours becomes 455.

In situations such as this when we're considering the use of a medication, the NNH needs to be balanced against the corresponding NNT summarizing the benefit of this treatment. The resulting crude "likelihood of being helped vs harmed" (LHH, see Ch. 4) by this treatment can provide the starting point for the last step, described in the next section. In Chapter 4, we outlined an approach to this in our discussion of a patient with dementia and explored the impact of use of antipsychotic medications on agitation AND mortality.

3. What are our patient's preferences, concerns and expectations from this treatment?

It is vital that we incorporate our patient's unique concerns and preferences into any shared decision-making process. In the case of potentially harmful therapy, just as in Chapter 4, we can ask our patient to quantify her values for both the potential adverse event(s) and the target event(s) we hope to prevent with the proposed therapy. The result is a severity-adjusted likelihood of being helped or harmed by the therapy. If we are unsure of our patient's baseline risk, or if she is unsure about her values for the outcomes, a sensitivity analysis can be done. That is, different values for relative severity could be inserted and we and our patient could determine at which point the decision would change.

4. What alternative treatments are available?

If this is a therapy under discussion, we and our patient could explore alternative management options. Is there another medication we could consider? Is there any effective non-pharmacological therapy available?

Returning to our patient and having reviewed the evidence about caffeine consumption and urge incontinence, she is considered to have heavy caffeine consumption. The bottom line from the study suggests that heavy caffeine consumption may increase the risk of detrusor instability but this association appears weak. However, after discussion with our patient, she would like to consider this option further in an attempt to reduce her symptoms and together we have outlined a proposal to look at an N-of-1 study to determine if a reduction in caffeine consumption will alleviate her symptoms (see Ch. 4 for detailed discussion of N-of-1 studies). She is also encouraged by the results of the small trials we found in which caffeine reduction (although part of multicomponent interventions) was found to decrease urinary symptoms. We have also discussed other risk factors that were identified in studies and that may be contributing to her incontinence including multiparity and history of forceps delivery. If no symptom resolution occurs with modification of caffeine consumption, we've agreed to consider a trial of pelvic floor muscle training which is a non-pharmacological intervention that has been proven to be beneficial in a systematic review.[11]

Practicing and teaching EBM in real-time 2

Formulating a question, and then retrieving, appraising and applying relevant evidence from the primary literature will usually take longer than the average clinical appointment. There are several ways to tackle the time constraints, focusing on finding shortcuts to facilitate practicing EBM. As we've already mentioned (in Ch. 2), if we can find our answer in a high-quality pre-appraised resource, we're ahead of the game – especially with a federated search. If we're lucky to have a local librarian or consultant pharmacist who can help us track down the evidence, we'd ask them for some help. (Although this requires that these team members have access to the evidence available online which isn't always the case in places where we've practiced!) Alternatively, we can share tasks with other colleagues, either locally or virtually using e-mail discussion groups or social networking sites. We'd also consider asking our patient to book a return visit in 1 week to review the evidence with them at that time, giving us some time to review the evidence between visits. If the same clinical issues arise commonly, we could find (e.g., in texts such as ACP PIER or *Clinical Evidence* or in non-commercial online services such as Medlineplus (http://medlineplus.gov) or develop our own patient information leaflets briefly summarizing some of the evidence. In the same way, we could keep our CATs (with expiry dates!) on file for our own needs if we expect the clinical problem to arise again. Depending on how interested our patient is in being part of the shared decision-making process, they could be involved in each step along the way. One resource that we've found useful in this process is DIPEx (www.healthtalkonline.org) (Fig. 7.2), which is a unique database of patient experiences that has been created through completion

7

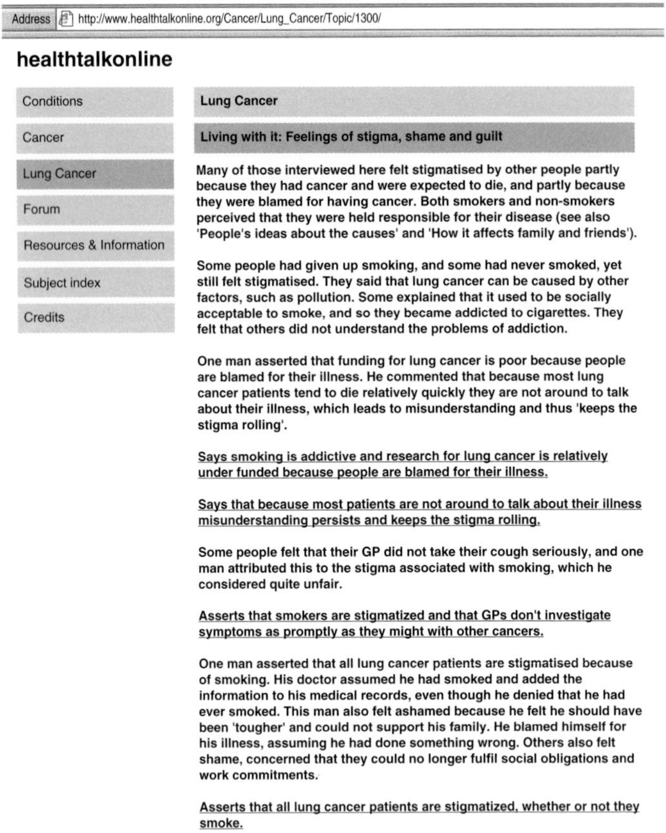

Address 🔲 http://www.healthtalkonline.org/Cancer/Lung_Cancer/Topic/1300/

healthtalkonline

Conditions	**Lung Cancer**
Cancer	**Living with it: Feelings of stigma, shame and guilt**
Lung Cancer	
Forum	
Resources & Information	
Subject index	
Credits	

Many of those interviewed here felt stigmatised by other people partly because they had cancer and were expected to die, and partly because they were blamed for having cancer. Both smokers and non-smokers perceived that they were held responsible for their disease (see also 'People's ideas about the causes' and 'How it affects family and friends').

Some people had given up smoking, and some had never smoked, yet still felt stigmatised. They said that lung cancer can be caused by other factors, such as pollution. Some explained that it used to be socially acceptable to smoke, and so they became addicted to cigarettes. They felt that others did not understand the problems of addiction.

One man asserted that funding for lung cancer is poor because people are blamed for their illness. He commented that because most lung cancer patients tend to die relatively quickly they are not around to talk about their illness, which leads to misunderstanding and thus 'keeps the stigma rolling'.

Says smoking is addictive and research for lung cancer is relatively under funded because people are blamed for their illness.

Says that because most patients are not around to talk about their illness misunderstanding persists and keeps the stigma rolling.

Some people felt that their GP did not take their cough seriously, and one man attributed this to the stigma associated with smoking, which he considered quite unfair.

Asserts that smokers are stigmatized and that GPs don't investigate symptoms as promptly as they might with other cancers.

One man asserted that all lung cancer patients are stigmatised because of smoking. His doctor assumed he had smoked and added the information to his medical records, even though he denied that he had ever smoked. This man also felt ashamed because he felt he should have been 'tougher' and could not support his family. He blamed himself for his illness, assuming he had done something wrong. Others also felt shame, concerned that they could no longer fulfil social obligations and work commitments.

Asserts that all lung cancer patients are stigmatized, whether or not they smoke.

Figure 7.2 Healthtalkonline screenshot.

of rigorous qualitative research. Patients' experiences with >40 health conditions are available on the site. A sibling site for adolescents is also available (www.youthhealthtalk.org).

Finally, we've found the James Lind Library (Fig. 7.3) (www.james-lindlibrary.org) to be a useful resource when we're teaching people to understand fair tests of treatments in healthcare. It is fun and useful because it provides examples of how a fair assessment should occur and

Address http://www.jameslindlibrary.org/trial_records/20th_Century/1960s/mcbride/mcbride_whole.html

Thalidomide and congenital abnormalities

Sir, — Congenital abnormalities are present in approximately 1.5% of babies. In recent months I have observed that the incidence of multiple severe abnormalities in babies delivered of women who were given the drug thalidomide ('Distaval') during pregnancy, as antiemetic or as a sedative, to be almost 20%. These abnormalities are present in structures developed from mesenchyme– i.e., the bones and the musculature of the gut. Bony development seems to be affected in a very striking manner, resulting in polydactyly, syndactyly, and failure of development of long bones, abnormally short femora and radii. Have any of your readers seen similar abnormalities in babies delivered of women who have taken this drug during pregnancy

Hurstville, New South Wales W.G McBride

In our issue of Dec. 2 we included a statement from the Distillers Company (Biochemicals) Ltd. Referring to "Reports from 2 overseas sources possibly associating thalidomide ('Distaval') With harmful effects on the foetus in early pregnancy". Pending further investigation, the company decided to withdraw from the market all its preparations containing thalidomide. – ED.L.

Figure 7.3 James Lind Library screenshot.

how these evaluations (randomized trials and systematic reviews) have evolved over time. Some material on this site relates to assessing benefits and harms including examples of "dramatic results", often about putative harm such as the one below.

References

1. Arya LA, Myers DL, Jackson ND. Dietary caffeine intake and the risk for detrusor instability: a case control study. *Obstet Gynecol.* 2000;96(1):85–89.
2. Onofrei MD, Butler KL, Fuke DC, et al. Safety of statin therapy in patients with preexisting liver disease. *Pharmacotherapy.* 2008;28(4):522–529.
3. Papanikolaou PN, Ioannidis HP. Availability of large-scale evidence on specific harms from systematic reviews of randomized trials. *Am J Med.* 2004;117(8):582–589.
4. Feinstein AR. ICD, POR, and DRG. Unsolved scientific problems in the nosology of clinical medicine. *Arch Intern Med.* 1988;148(10):2269–2274.
5. Zhan C, Miller MR. Administrative data based patient safety research: a critical review. *Qual Saf Health Care.* 2003;12(suppl II):ii58–ii63.

6. Doll R, Hill AB. The mortality of doctors in relation to their smoking habits; a preliminary report. *BMJ*. 1954;1(4877):1451–1455.

7. Doll R, Peto R, Boreham J, et al. Mortality in relation to smoking: 50 years' observations on male British doctors. *BMJ*. 2004;328(7455):1519.

8. Bernal-Delgado F, et al. The association between vasectomy and prostate cancer: a systematic review of the literature. *Fertil Steril*. 1998;70(2): 191–200.

9. Doll R, Hill AB. Mortality in relation to smoking: ten years' observations of British doctors. *BMJ*. 1964;1(5395):1399–1410.

10. Bryant CM, Dowell CJ, Fairbrother G. Caffeine reduction education to improve urinary symptoms. *Br J Nurs*. 2002;11(8):560–565.

11. Holroyd-Leduc J, Straus SE. Management of urinary incontinence in women: scientific review. *JAMA*. 2004;291(8):986–995.

Further reading

Guyatt G, Rennie D, Meade M, et al, eds.*Users' guides to the medical literature. A manual for evidence-based clinical practice*. Chicago: AMA press; 2008.

Haynes RB, Sackett DL, Guyatt GH, et al. *Clinical epidemiology: How to do clinical practice research*. Philadelphia: Lippincott Williams & Wilkins; 2006.

8 Evaluation

The fifth step in practicing EBM is self-evaluation and we'll suggest some approaches for doing that here. This book is geared to help individual clinicians to learn how to practice EBM so this section will mainly focus on how we can reflect on our own practice. However, some of us are also involved in teaching EBM and we've provided some tips on how to evaluate our teaching and additional relevant material is available on the accompanying CD. And, some clinicians, managers and policy-makers might be interested in evaluating how evidence-based practice is being implemented at a local, regional or national level and while this is not the aim of this book, we'll introduce this topic and point you to some useful resources for further information.

How am I doing?

This part of the chapter will describe the domains in which you might want to evaluate your performance. We also will note some aids to self-evaluation that you can find on the book's CD.

Evaluating our performance in asking answerable questions

Table 8.1 suggests some initial questions to consider about our own question-asking in practicing EBM. First, are we asking any questions at all? As our experience grows, are we using a map of where most questions come from (Table 1.2 is our version) to locate our knowledge gaps, and help us articulate questions? When we get stuck, are we increasingly able to get "unstuck" using the map or other devices? On a practical level, have we devised a method to note our questions as they occur, for later retrieval and answering when time permits? There are low-tech and high-tech options for this – some of us keep a logbook in our pocket to record our questions and the answers when we've had a chance to retrieve them. Alternatively, we could go for the high-tech option and use a program that we've devised for PDAs (available on the CD) that

---

Table 8.1 Self-evaluation in asking answerable questions

1. Am I asking any clinical questions at all?
2. Am I asking focused questions?
3. Am I using a "map" to locate my knowledge gaps and articulate questions?
4. Can I get myself "unstuck" when asking questions?
5. Do I have a working method to save my questions for later answering?

---

allows us to record our questions and answers. In some countries, this type of practice reflection is essential for maintaining certification from professional organizations.

Evaluating our performance in searching

Table 8.2 lists some questions we might want to ask ourselves about our performance in searching for the best evidence. Are we searching at all? Do we know the best sources of current evidence for our clinical discipline? Are we trying to find the highest quality evidence, aiming for the top of the "6s pyramid" as described in Chapter 2? Do we have access to the best evidence for our clinical discipline? Are the most crucial resources bookmarked? You might wish to try timing the steps in your search process: locating a resource, starting up the resource, typing in a question, getting the response, etc. Which of these can you speed up to become more efficient with this process? If we have started searching on our own, are we finding useful external evidence from a widening array of sources, and are we becoming more efficient in our searching? Are we using validated search filters when using MEDLINE? Are we using meta-search engines?

Table 8.2 A self-evaluation in finding the best external evidence

1. Am I searching at all?
2. Do I know the best sources of current evidence for my clinical discipline?
3. Do I have easy access to the best evidence for my clinical discipline?
4. Am I becoming more efficient in my searching?
5. Am I using truncations, Booleans, MeSH headings, thesaurus, limiters, and intelligent free text when searching MEDLINE?
6. How do my searches compare with those of research librarians or other respected colleagues who have a passion for providing best current patient care?

An efficient way of evaluating our searching skills is to ask research librarians or other respected colleagues to repeat a search that we've already done and then compare notes on both the searching strategy and the usefulness of the evidence we both found. Done this way, we benefit in three ways: from the evaluation itself, from the opportunity to learn how to do it better, and from the yield of additional external evidence on the clinical question that prompted our search. One thing we've found useful during Journal Club is to do a search in "real-time" and limit ourselves to 2 minutes for finding an answer to a clinical question. We then elicit feedback from colleagues on how we could improve the search the next time.

It might be wise to consult our nearest health sciences library about taking a course or personal tutorial, so that we can get to the level of expertise we need to carry out this second step in practicing EBM. We might even persuade one of the librarians to join our clinical team, an extraordinary way to increase our proficiency! We have found it very helpful to have a librarian join us (even occasionally) on clinical rounds; it's an opportunity for them to teach us searching tips as we try to become more efficient and effective searchers.

Evaluating our performance in critical appraisal

Table 8.3 lists some questions to examine how we're doing in critically appraising external evidence. Are we doing it at all? If not, can we identify the barriers to our performance and remove them? Once again, we might find that working as a member of a group (such as the Journal Club we describe in Ch. 9) could not only help us get going but also give us feedback about our performance.

Most clinicians find that critical appraisal of most types of articles becomes easier with time but find one or two that are more challenging. Again, this is a situation in which working in a group (even "virtual" groups) can quickly identify and resolve such confusion. Often in

8

Table 8.3 A self-evaluation in critically appraising the evidence for its validity and potential usefulness

1. Am I critically appraising external evidence at all?
2. Are the critical appraisal guides becoming easier for me to apply?
3. Am I becoming more accurate and efficient in applying some of the critical appraisal measures (such as likelihood ratios, NNTs and the like)?
4. Am I creating any appraisal summaries?

Journal Clubs we find that the focus is on therapy articles (we're often in our comfort zone with these articles) but one strategy we've found useful is to encourage participants to consider other study types and to engage in team learning. With team learning, the Journal Club is not resting on a single person appraising the article but instead it becomes a group activity. We can then proceed to consider whether we are becoming more accurate and efficient in applying some of the measures of effect (such as likelihood ratios, NNTs and the like). This could be done by comparing our results with those of colleagues who are appraising the same evidence, or by taking the raw data from an article abstracted in one of the journals of secondary publication, completing the calculations, and then comparing them with the abstract's conclusions. Another strategy to facilitate team-based appraisal is to provide half of the participants with an article that has found a positive result to an evaluation of a therapy, and the other half of the participants with an article that has found a different result from an evaluation of the same therapy. The two teams then discuss why such different results were obtained from the studies.

Finally, at the most advanced level, are we creating summaries of our appraisals? We could use formal CATMaker or GATE software to create these summaries or we could develop our own template for storing appraisals. We find CATMaker a useful teaching tool but often we find it too cumbersome for daily use in our clinical practice and instead we keep abbreviated versions of our appraisals using a simple template including the study citation, clinical bottom line, a 2-line description of the study methods and a brief table or summary of results. The CQ log allows us to create this database for our PDAs and is available on the book's website.

Evaluating our performance in integrating evidence and patients' values

Table 8.4 lists some elements of a self-evaluation of our skills in integrating our critical appraisals with our clinical expertise and applying the results in our clinical practice. We ask ourselves whether we are integrating our critical appraisals into our practice at all. Because the efforts we've expended in the previous three steps are largely wasted if we can't execute this fourth one, we'd need to do some soul-searching and carry out some major adjustments of how we spend our time and energy if we're not following through on it. Once again, talking with a mentor or working as a member of a group might help overcome this failure,

---

Table 8.4 A self-evaluation in integrating the critical appraisal with clinical expertise and applying the result in clinical practice

1. Am I integrating my critical appraisals into my practice at all?
2. Am I becoming more accurate and efficient in adjusting some of the critical appraisal measures to fit my individual patients (pre-test probabilities, NNT/f, etc.)?
3. Can I explain (and resolve) disagreements about management decisions in terms of this integration?

---

as might attending one of the EBM workshops. Once we are on track, we could ask ourselves whether we are becoming more accurate and efficient in adjusting some of the critical appraisal measures to fit our individual patients. Have we been able to find or otherwise establish pre-test probabilities that are appropriate to our patients and the disorders we commonly seek in them?

Are we becoming more adept at modifying measures like the NNT to take into account the "f" for our patient? One way to test our growing skills in this integration is to see whether we can use them to explain (and maybe even resolve!) disagreements about management decisions. We can do this among our colleagues in our practice or our residents on the teaching service.

Is our practice improving?

Although a self-evaluation showing success at the foregoing level should bring enormous satisfaction and pride to any clinician, we might want to proceed even further, and could ask ourselves whether what we have learned has been translated into better clinical practice (Table 8.5). While there are many, many frameworks that can be used to guide evidence implementation, we find the Knowledge to Action Framework is helpful

---

Table 8.5 A self-evaluation of changing practice behavior

1. When evidence suggests a change in practice, am I identifying barriers and facilitators to this change?
2. Have I identified a strategy to implement this change, targeted to the barriers I've identified?
3. Have I carried out any check, such as audits of my diagnostic, therapeutic, or other EBM performance including evidence use as well as impact on clinical outcomes?
4. Am I considering sustainability of this change?

8

when we are trying to implement evidence in our own practice.[1] This framework was based on a review of more than 30 theories of planned action and includes their common elements. Specifically, the framework includes assessing the gap in care (e.g., performing a chart audit to see if BMD tests are being ordered appropriately in our patients at high risk for osteoporotic fractures); adapting the evidence to the local context (e.g., determining what effective osteoporosis medications are available in our setting, at low/no cost to my patients); assessing the barriers and facilitators to evidence use (e.g., are BMD tests readily available? Do we need help in interpreting the results of BMD tests? Are our patients interested in considering osteoporosis medications? And, in some healthcare settings: Can our patients afford the test and, can our patients afford the medication(s)?); selecting an implementation strategy targeted to these barriers and facilitators (e.g., electronic reminders for physicians; patient information leaflet and web-based educational tool; insurance coverage for medications); evaluating evidence use (e.g., are BMDs being ordered appropriately? Are we prescribing osteoporosis medications for high risk patients?); monitoring outcomes (e.g., what is the fracture risk in our patients? What is their quality of life?) and assessing sustainability of evidence use (e.g., are we continuing to order BMDs and osteoporosis medication in relevant patients at 1 year, at 2 years, etc.?).

We think one of the most important steps in this process is to consider the barriers and facilitators to evidence use in our practice. Failing to do this step often results in failure of evidence implementation. Do we need new skills, equipment, organizational processes or a reminder system? For example, in one of our practices, we decided that diabetic patients should get annual foot checks including monofilament testing. To implement this, we needed the monofilaments, the skills to use them reliably, and a data entry field added to our annual check-up form as a reminder to test (and the result was a 50% reduction in unnecessary podiatry referrals).

Another important (but time consuming) piece in this process is to audit evidence uptake and its impact on clinical outcomes. Audits can tell us how we're doing as clinicians; and if we incorporate individualized feedback they can have a positive impact on our clinical performance. A bonus for completion is that many professional organizations provide CME credits for conducting them (although we don't see this as a reason to complete them!). Audits are much easier to perform if we have an electronic health record which allows us to capture the relevant data. However, most of us don't operate in paperless systems and thus we often have to rely on review of paper charts.

Audits can occur at various levels of complexity, and many hospitals have well-developed audit (or quality improvement) committees with full-time staff. Because this book is directed to individual clinicians, we won't devote space to audits carried out at these higher levels of organization. Practice audits are often carried out at a local, regional or national level and, attempts focused on how to change physician behavior at these levels. Several methods have been found to be effective, including academic detailing, opinion leaders and electronic reminders. As we've mentioned before, this is not the focus of this book and we refer you to some other resources listed at the end of this chapter which address this topic. Specifically, these resources focus on knowledge translation or implementation science, which is about putting evidence into practice at various levels within the healthcare system and not just at the level of the individual clinician–patient dyad which is the focus of this book.

If the audit shows that we've implemented the evidence, then we can celebrate and then perhaps consider how to improve further. If we haven't changed, rather than self-recriminations, we should ask what were the problems and barriers to change. Perhaps new barriers arose that required us to change our implementation strategy – in the complex healthcare environment, it is not unusual for this to happen! And thus, we re-enter the Knowledge-to-Action Cycle.

How much of our practice is evidence-based?

A number of clinical teams have looked at the extent to which practice is evidence-based. The impetus for their work was the "conventional wisdom" that only about 20% of clinical care was based in solid scientific evidence.* One of the first studies was performed on David Sackett's clinical service in Oxford, where at the time of their discharge, death, or retention in hospital at the end of the audited month, every patient was discussed at a team meeting and consensus reached on their primary diagnosis (the disease, syndrome, or condition entirely or, in the case of multiple diagnoses, most responsible for the patient's admission to hospital) and their primary intervention (the treatment or other maneuver that represented the most important attempt to cure, alleviate, or care for the primary diagnosis).[2] The primary intervention was then traced, either into an "instant resource book of evidence-based

8

---

*In 1963, the estimate was 9.3%. Forsyth G. An inquiry into the drug bill. Med Care 1963; 1: 10–16.

medicine" maintained by the consultant or to other sources (via computerized bibliographic database searching, into the published literature), and classified into one of three categories: interventions whose value (or non-value) is established in one or more randomized controlled trials or, better yet, systematic reviews of RCTs; interventions whose face-validity is so great that randomized trials assessing their value were unanimously judged by the team to be both unnecessary and, if they involved placebo treatments, unethical; and interventions in common use but failing to meet either of the preceding two criteria. Of the 109 patients diagnosed that month, 90 (82%) were judged by pre-set criteria to have received evidence-based interventions. The primary interventions for 53% of patients were based on one or more randomized trials or systematic reviews of trials. An additional 29% of patients received interventions unanimously judged to be based on convincing non-experimental evidence, and 18% received specific symptomatic and supportive care without substantial evidence that it was superior to some other intervention or to no intervention at all.

This audit confirmed that inpatient general medicine could be evidence-based and similar audits since then have been conducted in various settings around the world and in many different clinical disciplines including general surgery, hematology, child health, primary care, anesthesia and psychiatry. The truth is that most patients we encounter have one of just a few common problems, while the rare problems are thinly spread between many patients. As a result, searching for the evidence that underpins the common problems provides a greater and more useful reward for our effort than fruitless quests for evidence about problems we might encounter once a decade. That these studies have found evidence for the most common interventions has validated the feasibility of practicing EBM. The key point for readers of this book is to recognize how such audits not only focus on clinical issues that are central to providing high-quality evidence-based care but also provide a natural focus for day-to-day education, helping every member of the team keep up-to-date.

Evaluating our performance as teachers

We may be interested in evaluating our own EBM teaching skills or in evaluating an EBM workshop, or course. Table 8.6 lists some ways of evaluating how we're doing as teachers of EBM. When did we last issue an Educational Prescription (or have one issued to us)? If not at all, why not? Are we helping our trainees learn how to ask focused questions?

Table 8.6 A self-evaluation in teaching EBM

1. When did I last issue an educational prescription?
2. Am I helping my trainees learn how to ask focused questions?
3. Are we incorporating question asking and answering into everyday activities?
4. Are my learners writing educational prescriptions for me?
5. Am I teaching and modeling searching skills (and making sure that my trainees learn them)?
6. Am I teaching and modeling critical appraisal skills?
7. Am I teaching and modeling the generation of appraisal summaries?
8. Am I teaching and modeling the integration of best evidence with my clinical expertise and my patients' preferences?
9. Am I developing new ways of evaluating the effectiveness of my teaching?
10. Am I developing, sharing and/or evaluating EBM educational materials?

Are we teaching and modeling searching skills? Our time may be far too limited to provide this training ourselves, but we should be able to find some help for our learners and we should try to link them with our local librarians (again, if a librarian can join our clinical team, we can share the teaching). Are we teaching and modeling critical appraisal skills, and teaching and modeling the generation of appraisal summaries? Are we teaching and modeling the integration of best evidence with our clinical expertise and our patients' preferences? Are we developing new ways of evaluating the effectiveness of our teaching? Particularly important here are the development and use of strategies for obtaining feedback from our students and trainees about our skills and performance in practicing and modeling EBM. Finally, are we developing, sharing and/or evaluating EBM educational materials?

A very useful way of evaluating our performance is to ask our respected colleagues and mentors for feedback. We can invite our colleagues to join our clinical team or to view a video of our teaching performance and to discuss it with us afterward, giving us and them a chance to learn together. At some institutions, a teaching consultation service is available to observe our teaching and to provide us with constructive feedback. We might also seek out a workshop on EBM to refine our skills further.

8

Evaluations of strategies for teaching the steps of EBM

TM

Professional organizations and medical schools have moved from whether to teach EBM to how to teach EBM. And, therefore we might be interested in evaluating how EBM is taught in a course or at a workshop.

The next section will summarize evidence on strategies for teaching the elements of EBM. We'll use the "PICO" format for our discussion (see also Ch. 1).

Who are the "patients"?

Who are the targets for our clinical questions? Two groups can be readily identified: the clinicians who practice EBM and the patients they care for. There is an accumulating body of evidence relating to the impact of EBM on students and healthcare professionals. This ranges from systematic reviews of training in the skills of EBM to qualitative research describing the experience of EBM practitioners and barriers they've encountered to implementation. There is a paucity of evidence about the effect of EBM on patient care or patients' perceptions of their care but we are starting to see these outcomes being considered. We are also starting to see more educational interventions targeting the public and policy-makers.

What is the Intervention (and the control maneuver)?

Studies of the effect of teaching EBM are challenging to conduct because not only would they require large sample sizes and lengthy follow-up periods, but it's unethical to generate a comparison group of clinicians who'd be allowed to become out of date and ignorant of life-saving evidence accessible to and known by the evidence-based clinicians in the experimental group. Similarly it would be tough to get clinicians to agree to an evidence-poor teaching intervention!

In many studies of the impact of EBM, the intervention has proven difficult to define. It's unclear what the appropriate "dose" or "formulation" should be. Some studies use an approach to clinical practice while others use training in one of the discrete "microskills" of EBM such as MEDLINE searching or critical appraisal. Indeed, a review of graduate medical education in EBM found 18 reports of such curricula but the courses most commonly focused on critical appraisal skills, in many cases to the exclusion of other EBM skills.[3] Some studies looked at 90-minute workshops whereas others included courses that were held over several weeks to months. Since this review was published, more studies of EBM curricula have appeared in the literature including large group, small group, online and individual teaching sessions. These interventions have targeted various health care professionals including nurses, pharmacists, occupational therapists and physicians and different training levels including undergraduate, postgraduate and continuing education. Although the introduction of EBM into learning is underway, the challenge is to precede these changes with solid evidence that they will work. Although this challenge has rarely been set or met by previous architects of new curricula, we nonetheless have sought it here.

What are the relevant outcomes?

Effective EBM interventions will produce a wide range of outcomes. Changes in clinicians' knowledge and skills are relatively easy to detect and demonstrate. Changes in their behaviors and attitudes are harder to confirm, and as mentioned previously, changes in clinical outcomes, are even more challenging to detect. Accordingly, studies demonstrating better patient survival when practice is evidence-based (and worse when it is not) are at present, limited to the cohort "outcomes research" studies described in this book's Introduction.

As discussed above, the intervention has proven difficult to define and as a result, the evaluation of whether the intervention has met its goals has been challenging. In the Introduction, we outlined that not all clinicians want or need to learn how to practice all five steps of EBM. We discussed three potential methods for practicing EBM including the doing, using and replicating modes. "Doers" of EBM practice Steps 1–5, while "users" focus on searching for and applying pre-appraised evidence. And, "replicators" seek advice from colleagues who practice EBM. While all of us practice in these different modes at various times in our clinical work, our activity will likely fall predominantly into one of these categories. Most clinicians consider themselves users of EBM and surveys of clinicians show that only approximately 5% believe that learning the five steps of EBM was the most appropriate method for moving from opinion-based to evidence-based medicine.[4] The various EBM courses and workshops must therefore address the needs of these different learners. One size cannot fit all! And similarly, if a formal evaluation of the educational activity is required, the instruments used to evaluate whether we've helped our learners reach their goals should reflect the different learners and their goals. While there have been many questionnaires that have been shown to be useful in assessing EBM knowledge and skills, we must remember that the learners, knowledge and skills targeted by these tools may not be similar to our own. For those who are interested, we point you to the systematic review of instruments for evaluating education in evidence-based practice.[5] More than 104 evaluation instruments were identified with many of these having reasonable validity. This review highlighted gaps in the field of evaluation with most tools focusing on EBM skills and few tools focusing on assessing behaviors.

8

It should be noted that quite innovative methods of evaluation are being used as attention is moving from assessing not just EBM knowledge and skills but to behaviors, attitudes and clinical outcomes as well. For example, in a study evaluating an EBM curriculum in a family medicine training program, resident–patient interactions were videotaped and analyzed for EBM content.[6] EBM-OSCE stations have become standards in many medical schools and residency programs. In a high stakes certification exam in Canada, postgraduate trainees are tested on their ability to practice EBM with standardized patients and with clinical scenarios. Finally, some studies currently underway are measuring clinical outcomes.

1. Effects of teaching strategies on searching skills

Several studies have shown that we can improve searching skills. A randomized trial among first clinical year medical students showed that a 3-hour session on question formulation and database searching produced significant gains in the quality of evidence retrieved.[7] The failure of control students to gain these skills by "diffusion" means that these skills must be formally learnt. Similar improvements in searching MEDLINE, sustainable at up to 9 months of follow-up, have been found in postgraduate training programs.[8] And other studies have shown that while searching skills could be enhanced, some EBM interventions were unable to show impact on skill in applying the evidence to a clinical scenario.[9] An interesting study done by Ann McKibbon found that clinicians (when using their usual search resources) changed from a correct answer to a clinical question to an incorrect answer 10% of the time![10] However, participants often used search engines like Google to answer their questions, highlighting the need for us to include searching of appropriate evidence resources in educational curricula.

2. Effects of teaching strategies on critical appraisal skills

A review of seven studies that evaluated courses teaching critical appraisal skills showed gains in knowledge (as assessed by a written test) by undergraduates.[11] Postgraduates showed a smaller change in knowledge following a critical appraisal course. A Cochrane review found only one study that met the authors' inclusion criteria.[12] This study ($n=44$) found that a critical appraisal course increased knowledge of critical appraisal in the intervention group compared to the control group. Since this review was last updated in 2001, several additional studies have been published showing skills in critical appraisal of the literature can be enhanced.[13,14] We haven't been able to identify any studies that have looked at sustained use of medical literature over time.

3. Effects of teaching strategies on clinical decision-making

An undergraduate program adopting problem-based, self-directed learning around diagnosis and therapy has been shown to result in clinical clerks making more and better clinical decisions, which they are better able to defend than peers educated in a more conventional program.[15] Graduates of a problem-based medical school were found to be more up-to-date in the knowledge of the management of hypertension than graduates of a traditional curriculum.[16] In a before-and-after study, a multi-component EBM intervention including teaching EBM skills and provision of electronic resources to consultants and house-officers at a district general hospital found that the intervention significantly improved evidence-based practice patterns.[17]

Reports describing evidence-based rejuvenations of traditional educational events are growing exponentially (try searching Journal Clubs or teaching evidence-based medicine and see what comes up!), and case reports and a survey of US residency programs have concluded that the determinants of continuing high attendance at postgraduate Journal Clubs are mandatory attendance, the teaching of critical appraisal skills, emphasizing the primary literature, independence from faculty, and (big surprise!) free food![18,19] Journal Clubs have also been found to stimulate interest in research.[20] Finally, qualitative research has confirmed that teaching and learning critical appraisal are enjoyable, a fact that should not be underestimated in one's working life!

For those of you who have read this far, that's it, we're done! We hope you have enjoyed this book and its accompanying resources as well as learned from them, and we would appreciate your suggestions on how to make them more useful as well as more enjoyable.

Cheers.

8

References

1. Graham ID, Logan J, Harrison MB, et al. Lost in knowledge translation: time for a map? *J Contin Ed Health Prof.* 2006;26(1):13–24.

2. Ellis J, Mulligan I, Rowe J, et al. Inpatient general medicine is evidence-based. *Lancet.* 1995;346(8972):407–410.

3. Green ML. Graduate medical education training in clinical epidemiology, critical appraisal and evidence-based medicine: a critical review of curricula. *Acad Med*. 1999;74(6):686–694.

4. McColl A, Smith H, White P, et al. General practitioner's perceptions of the route to evidence-based medicine: a questionnaire survey. *BMJ*. 1998;316(7128):361–365.

5. Shaneyfelt T, Baum KD, Bell D, et al. Instruments for evaluating education in evidence-based practice. *JAMA*. 2006;296(9):1116–1127.

6. Ross R, Verdieck A. Introducing an evidence-based medicine curriculum into a family practice residency – is it effective? *Acad Med*. 2003;78(4):412–417.

7. Rosenberg W, Deeks J, Lusher A, et al. Improving searching skills and evidence retrieval. *J R Coll Physicians Lond*. 1998;32(6):557–563.

8. Smith CA, Ganschow P, Reilly BM, et al. Teaching residents evidence-based medicine skills. *JGIM*. 2000;15(10):710–715.

9. Kim S, Willett LR, Murphy DJ, et al. Impact of an evidence-based medicine curriculum on resident use of electronic resources: a randomised controlled study. *J Gen Intern Med*. 2008;23(11):1804–1808.

10. McKibbon KA, Fridsma DB. Effectiveness of clinician-selected electronic information resources for answering primary care physicians' information needs. *J Am Med Inform Assoc*. 2006;13(6):653–659.

11. Norman G, Shannon SI. Effectiveness of instruction in critical appraisal skills: a critical appraisal. *CMAJ*. 1998;158(2):177–181.

12. Parkes J, Hyde C, Deeks J, et al. Teaching critical appraisal skills in health care settings. *Cochrane Database Syst Rev*. 2001;(3): CD001270.

13. Krueger PM. Teaching critical appraisal: a pilot randomized controlled outcomes trial in undergraduate osteopathic medical education. *J Am Osteopath Assoc*. 2006;106(11):658–662.

14. Harewood GC, Hendrick LM. Prospective controlled assessment of the impact of formal evidence-based medicine teaching working on ability to appraise the medical literature. *Ir J Med Sci*. 2009; Aug 26. [Epub ahead of print].

15. Bennett K, Sackett DL, Haynes RB, et al. A controlled trial of teaching critical appraisal of the clinical literature to medical students. *JAMA*. 1987;257(18):2451–2454.

16. Shin JH, Haynes RB, Johnston M. Effect of problem-based, self-directed undergraduate education on lifelong learning. *CMAJ*. 1993;148(6):969–976.

17. Straus SE, Ball C, McAlister FA, et al. Teaching evidence-based medicine skills can change practice in a community hospital. *JGIM*. 2005;20(4):340–343.

18. Sidorov J. How are internal medicine residency journal clubs organized and what makes them successful? *Arch Int Med*. 1995;155(11):1193–1197.

19. Alguire PC. A review of journal clubs in postgraduate medical education. *JGIM*. 1998;13(5):347–353.

20. Moharari RS, Rahimi E, Najafi A, et al. Teaching critical appraisal and statistics in anaesthesia journal club. *QJM*. 2009;102(2):139–141.

Further reading

Davis D, Barnes B, Fox F, eds. *The continuing professional development of physicians: From research to practice*. Chicago: American Medical Association; 2003.

Straus SE, Tetroe J, Graham ID. *Knowledge translation in health care*. Oxford: Wiley/Blackwell/BMJ; 2009.

8

9 Teaching EBM

Throughout the book we've provided ideas for teaching methods when they fit with the themes of previous chapters (e.g., the Educational Prescription in Ch. 1) and you can find them in the index or by scanning the page margins for the mortar board icon. In this chapter, we've collected other ideas for teaching learners how to practice EBM. We'll describe three main modes for teaching EBM, consider some successes and failures with various teaching methods, and examine some specific clinical teaching situations.

We're clinical teachers and collectors of teaching methods, not educational theorists. From what we've learned so far about theories of learning, rather than adhering strictly to one theory we find ourselves using ideas and methods from several schools of thought. We collect here the lessons we've gathered about how to put these principles into practice, whether from our own experiences, from watching others, from the learning sciences, or from the emerging scholarship about what works in teaching EBM. In developing as teachers, we've been most strongly influenced by the people who taught us, yet we've also been influenced by several works on teaching and learning.[1-11]

Three modes of teaching EBM

From what we've done, seen, or heard about, we've noticed that although there may be as many ways to teach EBM as there are teachers, most of these methods fall into one of three categories or teaching modes: role modeling evidence-based practice, weaving evidence into teaching clinical medicine, and targeting specific EBM skills (Table 9.1).[12,13]

The first teaching mode involves role modeling the practice of EBM. For example, when you and a learner see together an ambulatory patient with asymptomatic, microscopic hematuria, you might ask yourself aloud a question about the frequency of underlying causes of this disorder, admit aloud you don't know the full answer, then find and appraise evidence about this topic, and discuss aloud how you'll use the evidence in

---

Table 9.1 Three modes of teaching EBM

1. Role modeling evidence-based practice:
   a. Learners see evidence as part of good patient care
   b. Teaching by example: "actions speak louder than words"
   c. Learners see us use judgment in integrating evidence into decisions
2. Weaving evidence into clinical teaching:
   a. Learners see evidence as part of good clinical learning
   b. Teaching by weaving: evidence is taught along with other knowledge
   c. Learners see us use judgment in integrating evidence with other knowledge
3. Targeting specific skills of evidence-based practice:
   a. Learners learn how to understand evidence and use it wisely
   b. Teaching by coaching: learners get explicitly coached as they develop
   c. Learners see us use judgment as we carry out the five EBM steps with them.

---

planning your diagnostic strategy. When we role model evidence-based practice, our learners see us incorporating evidence with other knowledge into clinical decisions. Learners come to see the use of evidence as part of good practice, not something separate from it. We show by our example that we really do it, when we really do it, and how we really do it. Since actions speak louder than words, we might expect role modeling to be among the more effective ways of teaching EBM, although as far as we know this hasn't been studied.

The second teaching mode involves weaving the results of clinical research with other knowledge you teach about a clinical topic. For instance, when you and a learner examine a patient with dyspnea, after teaching how to do percussion of the posterior thorax, you can summarize research results about this finding's accuracy and precision as a test for pleural effusion. When we include research evidence in what we teach about clinical medicine, our learners see us integrating evidence with knowledge from other sources – the biology of human health and disease, the medical humanities, the understanding of systems of healthcare, the values and preferences of patients, and our clinical expertise, to name a few. Thus, trainees come to see the use of evidence as part of good clinical learning, not something separate from it, all in the context of making real clinical decisions. We might expect this integration and vivid realism would make weaving evidence into clinical teaching to be another very effective teaching mode, although we haven't seen this studied either.

The third mode involves targeted teaching of the skills of evidence-based practice. For instance, when learning about the care of a patient facing newly diagnosed lymphoma, in addition to teaching the "content" of this cancer's prognosis, you can also teach your team members the "process" of how to find and critically appraise studies of prognosis. When we target the skills of EBM, we help our learners build their capacity to independently develop and maintain their clinical competence. Learners come to see using EBM skills as part of lifelong professional development, not an isolated classroom exercise. The Cochrane review found some trial evidence that teaching critical appraisal improves participants' knowledge but no trial evidence about which methods are most effective.[14] Also, a before–after study found that teaching EBM skills to trainees in a community hospital led to improvements in the processes of patient care.[15]

We use all three modes of teaching EBM, moving from one to another to fit the clinical and teaching circumstances. Each mode requires different preparation and skills, so we may begin our teaching careers feeling more comfortable with one mode than the others. Yet, since good teachers of EBM (or anything else for that matter) are made, not born, with deliberate practice of and purposeful reflection on each mode we can refine both our skills with each mode and in blending all three.[11] We find that conscientiously using evidence in our practice and teaching (Modes 1 and 2) gives us more authenticity to our learners when we teach them about specific EBM skills (Mode 3).

Teaching EBM: top 10 successes

Reflecting on what worked well can help us refine our teaching.[16] Here we collect 10 characteristics we've noticed when teaching EBM has worked well.

1. When it centers around real clinical decisions and actions

Since practicing EBM begins and ends with patients, it shouldn't surprise you that our most enduring and successful efforts in teaching EBM have been those that centered on the illnesses of patients directly under the care of our learners. The clinical needs of these patients serve as the starting point for identifying our knowledge needs and asking answerable clinical questions that are directly relevant to those needs. By returning to our patients' problems after searching and appraising evidence about them, we can demonstrate how to integrate evidence with other knowledge and our patients' preferences and unique circumstances. When targeting EBM skills in Mode 3, if the learning group members are not on the same clinical service and don't share responsibility for the same patients, we can still engage the group in discussing one or more real clinical decisions they've either faced already or expect to face in the future. By centering our teaching around the care of

9

either current or future patients, our trainees learn how to use evidence in its natural context: thus informing real decisions and actions.

2. When it focuses on learners' actual learning needs

We think teaching means helping learners learn, and we think of ourselves as guides or coaches of learning. Since clinical learners will vary widely in their motivations, their starting knowledge, their learning prowess and skills, their learning contexts and available time for learning, we may need to employ a variety of teaching strategies and tactics. One size does not fit all, so in our teaching practices we need the skills to accurately assess our learners' developmental stage, diagnose their learning needs, and select appropriate teaching interventions. We need to be patient with our learners, adjusting our teaching to match their developmental stage and the pace of their understanding. Since many of our learners will also have externally imposed demands they must satisfy, like passing written exams, we need to acknowledge these conflicting demands, help learners cope with them, and adjust our teaching to fit the circumstances.

3. When it balances passive ("diastolic") with active ("systolic") learning

Learning clinical medicine has been described using an analogy to the cardiac cycle, with passive learning devices like listening to a lecture compared with diastolic filling and active learning devices compared with systolic pumping.[17] Just as with the phases of the cardiac cycle, both kinds of learning are useful, and both work best when used in balance with each other. Passive techniques may be effective for learning some kinds of knowledge (the "know what"), yet only through active methods can we learn how to put this knowledge into action (the "know how"). Recent reviews of comparative studies in science curricula suggest that using active and inductive learning strategies helps students achieve higher test scores and other improvements, when compared with students using passive approaches.[18,19] Since most trainees arrive onto our clinical teams having had much more experience with passive learning than active,[20] to help restore balance we find ourselves strongly emphasizing active learning strategies.

4. When it connects "new" knowledge to "old" (what learners already know)

By the time they arrive onto our clinical teams, most of our learners have very large funds of knowledge, of both experiential and book learning. Whether teaching in Modes 1, 2, or 3, with questions we can stimulate learners to recall knowledge from their memories, which activates this knowledge for use and helps us identify any knowledge gaps or misunderstandings. By connecting the new information we teach to their existing knowledge networks, we help learners to better comprehend the new lessons and put them into context. We also help learners reorganize their knowledge into schemes more useful for clinical decision-making.

5. When it involves everyone on the team

When learners join our clinical teams, they join two co-existing communities.[9] By sharing the responsibility for the care of the team's patients, they join a "community of practice" that faces the same clinical problems and works together toward their solutions. By sharing the responsibility to learn whatever is needed for sound clinical decisions, they join a "community of learning" that faces common learning challenges and works together to meet them. These two communities don't just co-exist, they interact. The shared work makes the learning necessary and useful, and the shared learning informs the team's clinical decisions and actions.[9] New students may be unfamiliar with working in these communities, so their seniors need to orient them as they join. When we as teachers divide the work of learning into chunks so that everyone can be involved, we help the team in four ways. First, a broader range of questions can be asked and answered, since the work can be shared by several people. Second, when seniors pair up with juniors to help them track down and appraise answers, their capacity for teamwork is reinforced. Third, since every team member can benefit from each team member's efforts, sharing lessons across the team multiplies the learning yields. Fourth, the team's interactive discussions as they learn can help individual team members clarify misconceptions, consolidate the lessons learned, and consider their implications for decision and action. Involving everyone needn't mean that all are assigned equal amounts of work – Educational Prescriptions (Ch. 1) can be handed out in differing amounts depending on workloads.

6. When it attends to all four domains of learning: affective, cognitive, conative, and psychomotor

First, as we mentioned in Chapter 1, learning can involve strong emotions, whether "positive", such as the joy of discovery or the fun of learning with others, or "negative", such as the fear of being asked a question, the shame of not knowing an answer, or the anger when learning time is squandered.

We can help learners grow in the affective domain of learning by helping them acknowledge the feelings of learning and developing appropriate, rather than maladaptive, responses (Modes 2 and 3). We can also help learners by showing some of our own feelings, such as our enthusiasm for learning (Mode 1). Second, recall that making sound clinical decisions requires us to recall, think with, and make judgments about several different kinds of knowledge, developed through different ways of knowing – we develop clinical expertise through experience with patient care and with coaching, we develop knowledge of our patients' perspectives and preferences through conversation and working with them, while we develop knowledge of research results through reading and critical appraisal. We can help our learners grow in the cognitive domain of learning by identifying these different sources of knowledge as we teach (Mode 2), and by coaching them to refine their abilities to know and learn in each way (Mode 3). Third, learning evidence-based practice involves translating knowledge into action, and the commitment and drive to perform these actions to the best of our abilities. This disposition to act for the benefit of others, combining ethical principles with the striving for excellence and pride in our work, has been termed the conative domain of learning.[21] We can help our learners grow in this conative domain by our actions, wherein we show our striving to improve and we demonstrate the pragmatics of how to turn new learning into better doing (Mode 1). We can also coach our learners on such things as assessing their own performance and developing plans for change (Mode 3). Fourth, learning EBM involves some physical actions, including practical tasks like capturing our questions to answer, using search interfaces, and so forth. We can help our learners grow in this psychomotor domain both by role-modeling (Mode 1), so our learners see what the actions look like when done well, and by explicit coaching (Mode 3), so they get feedback on how they are doing and how to improve.

7. When it matches, and takes advantage of, the clinical setting, available time, and other circumstances

Each patient situation and clinical setting define a different learning context, where things like the severity of illness, the pace of the work, the available time and person-power all combine to determine what can be learned and when, where, how and by whom it is learned. Teaching tactics that work well in one setting (e.g., the outpatient clinic) may not fit at all in other settings (e.g., the intensive care unit). We can improve patient- and learner-centered learning by capitalizing on opportunities that present themselves in these different settings *as they occur*, using a mix of Modes 1 and 2.

8. When it balances preparedness with opportunism

Just because teaching EBM in Modes 1 or 2 may start and end with today's patient, that doesn't mean it can't be well prepared. Instead, we can anticipate many of the questions our learners will ask, since they'll arise from the patients, health states, and clinical decisions we encounter frequently in our practice and teaching settings. To prepare for these opportunities, we can gather, appraise and summarize the evidence we'll use to inform those decisions, and then place these summaries at or near the sites of care. We need only recognize the clinical situations when (not if) they occur, seize the teaching moment and guide the learners in understanding and using the evidence. This kind of opportunism can be supplemented by another kind – recognizing teaching opportunities among questions for which we haven't prepared ahead; to model and involve learners in the steps of asking questions, finding and appraising evidence, and integrating it into our clinical decisions.

9. When it makes explicit how to make judgments, whether about the evidence itself or about how to integrate evidence with other knowledge, clinical expertise and patient preferences and circumstances

Practicing EBM requires us to use judgment when choosing questions, when selecting knowledge resources, when appraising evidence critically, and when integrating the evidence into clinical decisions. Using judgment requires not only that we are be able to sort, weigh, and integrate knowledge of different kinds, but also that we can reflect on the underlying values made visible by our choices. Learning to make these judgments wisely takes time and practice, so it seems sensible to have our learners spend this time well by making this practice deliberate and these discussions explicit. While medical educational research may not yet have confirmed the value of such an explicit, reflective (also termed "meta-cognitive") approach, we reckon that the opposite strategy, that of ignoring judgment and abandoning our learners in their quest to develop it, is both ineffective and irresponsible. Thus, when we're teaching in Modes 1, 2, or 3, we use an explicit approach in guiding learners through clinical decisions.

10. When it builds learners' lifelong learning abilities

Clinical practice can be thought of as the ultimate open-book test, occurring daily over a lifetime of practice, with the world's knowledge potentially available as "the book" for clinicians to use. To develop and sustain the skills to use this knowledge wisely, learners need hard work and coaching, concentrating on such things as reflection, to recognize their own learning needs; resilience, to respond adaptively to their cognitive dissonance; and resourcefulness, to know how to carry out learning on their own.[6] One method to stimulate this process is to make learning multi-staged. When we divide the learning into manageable chunks and plan its achievement over several stages, we allow learners to try their hands at each stage, coming to the next encounter with both the learning yield and with experiences that can guide new learning objectives. Multi-staged learning also helps with managing time well, because on busy clinical services, it is usually easier to schedule several short appointments for learning rather than one large block. Multi-staged learning allows learning to be "vertically aligned", meaning that when we return later to the same material, we can reinforce what was learned before and then add new material appropriate to our learners' advancing skills.

Teaching EBM: top 10 failures

To compare with these successes, we collect here 10 mistakes we've either made or seen in teaching EBM, since reflecting on failures can also help refine one's teaching.[22]

1. When learning how to do research is emphasized over *how to use* it

2. When learning how to do statistics is emphasized over *how to interpret* them

These first two mistakes happen when experts in any field of basic science hold the notion that in order to pragmatically apply the fruits of a science, learners have to master its methods of inquiry. This is demonstrably untrue (doctors save the lives of patients with heart failure by prescribing them beta-blockers, not by learning how to measure the number of beta-receptors in cardiac muscle cells). It is also counterproductive, for it requires learners who want to become clinicians to learn the skills of transparently foreign careers, and we shouldn't be surprised by learners' indifference and hostility to courses in statistics and epidemiology. Our recognition of these mistakes explains why there is so little about statistics in this book and why our emphasis throughout is on how to use research reports, not how to generate them.

3. When teaching EBM is limited only to finding flaws in published research

4. When teaching portrays EBM as substituting research evidence for, rather than adding it to, clinical expertise, patient values and circumstances

These mistakes can occur when any narrow portion of a complex undertaking is inappropriately emphasized to the exclusion of all other portions. In response, learners may develop skills in one step of EBM, such as the ability to find study flaws in critical appraisal, but don't develop any other skills. This hurts learners in two ways. First, by seeing an unbalanced approach to appraising evidence, learners can develop protracted nihilism, a powerful *de*-motivator of evidence-based learning. Second, without learning to follow critical appraisal by integrating evidence sensibly into clinical decisions, learners aren't prepared to act independently on evidence in the future (when their teachers are gone), so they remain dependent on others to interpret evidence for them and tell them how to act.

5. When teaching with or about evidence is disconnected from the team's learning needs about either their patients' illnesses or their own clinical skills

This mistake can happen in several ways, such as when we fail to begin and end our teaching sessions with the learners' patients; when we fail to diagnose either the patients' clinical needs or our learners' resulting learning needs; or when we fail to connect our teaching to our learners' motivations, career plans or stage of development as clinicians. The resulting disconnection between what we teach and what the learners need to learn usually means not only that the learners won't retain anything we do cover, but also that we consume the available learning time before they can learn what they really need to know. As such foregone learning opportunities accumulate, our learners fall behind their peers in developing clinical excellence and lifelong learning skills.

9

6. When the amount of teaching exceeds the available time or the learners' attention

7. When teaching occurs at the speed of the teacher's speech or mouse clicks, rather than at the pace of the learners' understanding

These two mistakes occur when the teacher overestimates the amount that should be covered in the available time. Although teachers' motives needn't be evil – these mistakes can arise simply out of enthusiasm for the subject – the resulting overly long and/or overly fast presentation taxes the learners' abilities to register, comprehend, or retain the material covered. For example, at a recent lecture, the speaker showed 96 visually complex slides while talking rapidly for all of the allotted 30 minutes, leaving listeners unable to decode the graphs on one slide before the next was shown, resulting in more of a "shock and awe campaign" than a useful learning experience.

8. When the teacher strives for full educational closure by the end of each session, rather than leaving plenty to think about and learn between sessions

The eighth mistake happens when we behave as if learning only occurs during formal teaching sessions. This behavior is harmful in two ways. First, it cuts off problem-solving during the sessions themselves ("We're running out of time, so I want to stop this discussion and give you the right answers"). Second, it prevents or impairs the development of the self-directed learning skills that will be essential for our learners' continuing professional development.

9. When it humiliates learners for not already knowing the "right" fact or answer

10. When it bullies learners to decide or act based on fear of others' authority or power, rather than based on authoritative evidence and rational argument

These entries are included here because they are still commonplace among medical education programs, and at some of these institutions they remain a source of twisted pride. Such treatment of learners by their teachers is not simply wrong in human terms, it is counterproductive. First, the resulting shame and humiliation learners feel will strongly discourage the very learning that the teacher's ridicule was meant to stimulate.[23] Second, in adapting to the rapid loss of trust and safety in the learning climate, learners will start employing strategies to hide their true learning needs and protect themselves from their teachers, undermining future learning and teaching efforts. Understandably, learners with prior experiences of these behaviors may be very reluctant to even start the practice of EBM by asking a question, since it exposes them to the potential threat of repeated abuse. Contrast this with the actions of colleague David Pencheon who asks new medical students questions of increasing difficulty until they respond with "I don't know" Upon hearing these words, he rewards them with a box of candy and tells them that these are the three most important words in medicine.[24]

Having considered these successes and failures, we'll turn to ways to incorporate teaching EBM into some learning encounters that are commonly present in the education of clinicians in many countries. We'll explore two of these opportunities in detail.

Teaching and learning EBM on an inpatient service

Hospitals comprise several different clinical settings, such as general or specialty wards, intensive care units and emergency departments, each with their own opportunities and challenges for learning and teaching.[25] Yet across hospital settings, there are several common types of teaching rounds, seven of which we've summarized in Table 9.2. Although they differ, these rounds share several features, including severe constraints on learners' time and the innumerable interruptions. Little surprise, then, that for most of these types of rounds, much of our EBM teaching is by Modes 1 and 2, modeling evidence-based practice and weaving evidence into teaching clinical topics, rather than by Mode 3.

We hope that Table 9.2 is self-explanatory, and will confine this text to describing the EBM strategies and resources that we use during them. During rounds on newly admitted patients ("post-take" or "admission" rounds), there is usually time only for quick demonstrations of evidence-based bits of the clinical exam and how to get from pre-test to post-test probabilities of the leading diagnosis (in about 2–5 min), or for introducing concise (1 page or 2–4 PDA screens) and instantly available (within <15 seconds) synopses of evidence about the key diagnostic and treatment decisions that have been, are being, or ought to be carried out.

Can synopses of evidence really get there that fast? Yes, by using either or both of two strategies: first, anticipate the clinical decisions you're likely to encounter, then find (or make) concise synopses of the evidence that

9

Table 9.2 Incorporating EBM into inpatient rounds

Type of round	Objectives[a]	Evidence of highest relevance	Restrictions[b]	Strategies
"Post-take" or admission rounds (after every period on-call, all over the hospital, by post-call team and consultant)	Decide on working diagnosis and initial therapy of newly admitted patients	Accuracy and precision of the clinical examination and other diagnostic tests; efficacy and safety of initial therapy	Time, motion (can't stay in one spot), and fatigue of team post-call	Demonstrate evidence-based (EB) exam and getting from pre-test to post-test probability; carry a PDA or a loose-leaf book with synopses of evidence; write educational prescriptions; add a clinical librarian to the team
Morning Report (every day, sitting down with entire medical service)	Briefly review new patients and discuss and debate the process of evaluating and managing one or more of them	Accuracy and precision of the clinical examination and other diagnostic tests; efficacy and safety of initial therapy	Time	Educational Prescriptions for foreground questions (and Fact follow-ups for background questions); give 1–2 min summaries of critical appraisal topics
Work rounds (every day, on one or several wards, by trainees)	Examine every patient and determine their current clinical state; review and (re)order tests and treatments	Accuracy and precision of diagnostic tests; efficacy and safety of ongoing Rx, and interactions	Time and motion	In electronic records, create links between test results or Rx orders and the relevant evidence
Consultant walking rounds (1–3 times a week, on one or several wards, by trainees and consultant)	As in work rounds, but objectives vary widely by consultant	As in work rounds, plus those resulting from individual consultant's objectives	Time, relevance to junior members ("shifting dullness")	Model how to explain evidence to patients and incorporate into decisions (e.g., LHH)

Review rounds (or "card flip") (every day, sitting down and at the bedside, by trainees and consultants)	45 second reviews of each patient's diagnosis, Rx, progress, and discharge plans; identification of complicated patients who require bedside exam and more discussion	Wherever the educational prescriptions have led the learners	Time	Educational Prescriptions for foreground questions (and Fact follow-ups for background questions); give 1–2 min summaries of critical appraisal; audit whether you are following through on EB care
Social issues rounds (periodically, by trainees and a host of other professionals)	Review of each patient's status, discharge plan, referral, and post-hospital follow-up	Efficacy and safety of community services and social interventions	Time, availability of relevant participants, and enormous burden of paperwork	Ask other health professionals to provide synopses of evidence for what they routinely propose
Preceptor rounds ("pure education") (1–2 times a week, by learners (often stratified) and teacher)	Develop and improve skills for clinical examination and presentation	Accuracy and precision of the clinical examination	Time, teacher's energy and other commitments	Practice presentations and feedback; use evidence about clinical exam; Educational Prescriptions for foreground questions (and Fact follow-ups for background questions); give concise summaries on critical appraisal
"Down time" or "dead space" during any round	Wait for the elevator or for a report or for a team member to show up, catch up, answer a page, get off the phone, find a chart, etc.	No limit	Imagination and ingenuity	Insert synopses of evidence, either from recent Educational Prescriptions (and fact follow-ups), or from pre-appraised evidence resources

a Increasingly, all rounds include the objective of discharging patients as soon as possible.
b All rounds require confidentiality when discussions of individual patients occur in public areas.

9

can inform those decisions and carry them with you. We've seen several formats used, including structured synopses on paper in a binder (Dave Sackett carried his "Big Red Book") [26], on notebook computer carried by a cart [27], in concise summaries carried in a PDA,[28] and both summaries and articles stored on a portable USB flash drive. Second, as information technology advances, more of us may find ourselves working in health systems that provide instant electronic access to evidence resources (as outlined in Ch. 2). When the evidence isn't so quickly to hand, we can write Educational Prescriptions to be filled after admission rounds, as we described in Chapter 1. In many centers, the individual teams' post-take rounds are supplemented by a service-wide, sit-down "Morning Report". Since not every admission needs to be discussed, this round can focus on patients who have the most to teach us.

"Work rounds", during which the team's trainees carry out the rapid, detailed, bedside review of patients' problems and progress and the review and ordering of their diagnostic tests and treatments, provide a challenging, yet fruitful setting for teaching in Modes 1 or 2. Most challenging perhaps is that the consultant/attending teacher is not present, yet the teacher can still influence the team's learning during these rounds, using the following three strategies: first, once the team has adopted the approach of integrating evidence into decisions when the attending is present, we can encourage its continued use by debriefing them on their successes and failures in applying evidence to decisions, and on questions they'd posed during work rounds, and by helping them to find evidence-based answers the whole team can use. Second, we can help our entire team get access to the evidence synopses we use when we are there, either by sharing them (e.g., handing them a one-page paper synopsis or "beaming" from our PDA to theirs) or by showing them how to access the resources themselves (e.g., providing URLs for filtered resources). Third, in some centers, the information systems that record patients' clinical, test and treatment data are being linked to electronic, "pop up" guidelines or summaries of evidence that can help team members take appropriate action.

"Consultant walking rounds" provide an excellent opportunity for the consultant to model how to combine evidence with patients' values and expectations in making management decisions. For example, the consultant might take 5–10 minutes to demonstrate how to use the likelihood of being helped vs harmed (LHH) by a treatment under consideration (as we showed you in Chapter 4). These rounds also provide great opportunities to teach in Mode 2, for example, by incorporating evidence about the accuracy of findings of volume depletion along with teaching how to choose the initial intravenous fluid for a patient with hypovolemia.

Many consultants (some of whom still keep note cards on each patient) lead short (<1 h), frequent (e.g., daily, when not "on take") "review rounds" (sometimes called the "card flip") of all patients on the service. This has been most fruitful for us when we held it in a work/seminar room right on or near the wards. Patients are summarized in four quick phrases (what they've got, what we're doing about it, how they are doing, when and where they are going), and this quick review is interrupted for only two reasons. The first reason is when a patient is so sick or unstable or so problematic that he or she needs to be examined by the whole team. The second interruption is for evidence-based learning. These may be precipitated by any team member and are of three types: first, challenges to provide evidence that the evaluation or management decisions being made for a patient are valid and appropriate; second, quick responses, usually with evidence synopses, to earlier challenges from previous rounds; and third, very brief demonstrations of the critical appraisal or application of evidence to specific patients.

' "Pure" education rounds' are conducted after the patients have been cared for, and enjoy the luxuries of relaxed time and choice of topic. Topics of relevance to EBM include thorough bedside evaluations of the techniques, accuracy and precision of the clinical examination; detailed learner-led discussions of how they found and appraised evidence; and detailed explanation and practice of skills such as generating patient-specific NNTs and NNHs. When these rounds are directed to new clinical clerks, they can include mastery of the orderly, thorough presentation of patients on the service, along the lines shown in Table 9.3.

Finally, all rounds of teams of size n are peppered with "down times" or "dead spaces" that interrupt the learning process and annoy at least $(n-1)$ of its members. Rather than permit learning to decelerate or be replaced by thoughts of lunch and sore backs, teachers can seize the moment and insert narrow "slices" of evidence, instead of the "whole pie",[29] from a recent evidence-based journal or website visit, or perhaps from a previously prepared evidence synopsis. Because no learner wants to be excluded from receiving these learning slices, this tactic encourages team members to avoid causing future down time.

Teaching and learning EBM in the outpatient clinic

Time both hampers and favors teaching in the outpatient setting. On the one hand, individual outpatient appointments are short, constraining both the number and breadth of clinical and learning issues that can be addressed during any single visit.[30] On the other hand, outpatient

---

Table 9.3 A guide for learners presenting an "old" patient at follow-up rounds

The presentation should summarize 20 things in 2 min:
1. The patient's name
2. The patient's age
3. The patient's sex
4. The patient's occupation/social role
5. When the patient was admitted (or transferred) to the service
6. The clinical problem(s) that led to admission (or transfer). (A clinical problem can be a symptom, a sign, a cluster of symptoms and signs, a clinical syndrome, an event, an injury, a test result, a diagnosis, a psychologic state, a social predicament, etc.)
7. The number of active problems the patient has at present

For each active problem:
8. Its most important symptoms, if any
9. Its most important signs, if any
10. The results of diagnostic tests or other evaluations
11. The explanation (diagnosis or health state) for the problem
12. The treatment plan instituted for the problem
13. The response to this treatment plan
14. The future and contingency plans for this problem

(Repeat 8–14 for each active problem)
15. Your plans for discharge, post-hospital care, and follow-up
16. Whether you've filled the Fact follow-up or Educational Prescription that you requested when this patient was admitted (in order to better understand the background of this patient's condition or the foreground of how best to care for this patient, respectively)

If so:
17. How you found the relevant evidence
18. What you found: the clinical bottom line from that evidence
19. Your critical appraisal of that evidence for its validity, importance, and applicability
20. How that critically appraised evidence will alter your care of that (or the next similar) patient.

If not:
17a. When you are going to fill the Fact follow-up or Educational Prescription.

---

illnesses and their care typically occur over more than one visit, often over months or even years, thereby providing lengthy interludes for extensive learning.[31] Just as with inpatient services, the outpatient setting is particularly well suited to teaching in Modes 1 and 2, role modeling and interweaving evidence with other topics. The types of rounds that occur in outpatient areas are summarized in Table 9.4.

Table 9.4 Incorporating EBM into outpatient rounds

Type of round	Objectives	Evidence of highest relevance	Restrictions[a]	Strategies
Clinic conference (before or after each half-day session, by small groups of learners and attendings)	Review the diagnosis and management of common outpatient disorders	Manifestations of disease, differential diagnosis, pre-test probability, accuracy and precision of diagnostic tests, efficacy and safety of Rx	Time, tardiness, and duties elsewhere	Educational Prescriptions for foreground questions (and Fact follow-ups for background questions); use, make or update concise summaries of evidence, such as CATs
Preceptorship during initial visits	Decide on working diagnosis and therapy	Accuracy and precision of clinical exam and diagnostic tests; efficacy and safety of initial therapy	Time, incomplete information	Demonstrate evidence-based (EB) exam and getting from pre-test to post-test probability; provide preassembled evidence summaries on diagnostic tests and initial Rx; write Educational Prescriptions
Preceptorship during follow-up visits	Review current status and adjust ongoing therapy	Long-term prognosis; efficacy and safety of alternative treatment options; harms from treatment	Time and changing patient needs	Model incorporation of patients' values, e.g., using LHH; fill Educational Prescriptions
Ambulatory Morning Report	Review case of particular outpatient(s)	Anything; most common are diagnostic tests and treatment options	Time; interruptions; widely varying levels of experience	Hold session in room with access to evidence resources; write and fill Educational Prescriptions; review old and new evidence summaries; give 1-min summaries on critical appraisal, NNT, etc.

[a]All rounds require confidentiality when discussions of individual patients occur in public areas.

9

237

The "clinic conferences", typically devoted to reviewing the diagnosis and management of common outpatient disorders, can abandon passive annual lectures and devote themselves to reviewing and discussing new evidence that guides key clinical decisions for these conditions, emphasizing the use of pre-appraised or filtered resources. Participants can make concise summaries of the evidence, or review and update the prior years' versions, then store these summaries nearby for ongoing use in their practices. Active learning occurs, and senior trainees can be asked to help their junior colleagues "learn the ropes" of how to take part in these processes.

Initial outpatient visits share objectives and constraints with "post-take" rounds on new inpatient admissions, so the same strategies apply. These are quick demonstrations of evidence-based bits of the clinical exam and how to get from pre-test to post-test probabilities of the initial diagnosis, plus instantly available (<15 seconds) evidence about key diagnostic and treatment decisions that have been, are being, or ought to be carried out.

Follow-up visits usually occur long enough after initial visits to allow learners to accomplish substantial problem-based learning between visits that can even be in multiple stages. When the learner first encounters an ambulatory patient, the teacher can coach them on the process of asking an answerable clinical question about one of the patient's problems and writing an educational prescription. At subsequent clinic sessions (and before the patient's follow-up visit), the teacher can review the learner's search strategies and critical appraisal of the evidence found. At the time of patient follow-up, the teacher and the learner can discuss how to integrate the evidence into clinical decisions and actions. The learner can then be asked to write a concise summary of the evidence, which the teacher and learner can review at another clinical session. Learning in this way doesn't take long at each stage (usually <5 min), yet over time leads to cumulative development of EBM skills.

Finally, some teaching outpatient departments hold "Morning Reports" similar to those held on the inpatient service. They labor under the same restrictions, but also offer the same rich variety of opportunities for teaching and learning.

Writing structured summaries of evidence-based learning episodes

At several points in the above discussion, we've mentioned the idea of writing or using a structured summary of evidence to aid our learning. Over the years, we've used or heard about several different structures, but the one we find ourselves using most often is the Critically

Appraised Topic, or CAT (Table 9.5). A CAT is a structured, one-page summary of the results of an evidence-based learning effort, in which a patient's illness stimulates a learner's question, for which the learner finds evidence, appraises the evidence, and decides whether and how to use that evidence in the care of the patient.[32] Because of its "quick and dirty" nature, a CAT may have limitations. The evidence found and selected for use may not be all there is, or even the best there is (a CAT is *not* a systematic review). Because the emphasis is on whether and how to use the evidence in one's own practice setting, the CAT may or may not apply to many or even any other settings (a CAT is *not* a practice guideline). A CAT might contain errors of calculation or appraisal judgments, and is thus not guaranteed to be error-free or permanent.

Despite these limitations, we find writing CATs helps us in four ways: first, writing down on one page the question, the answer, and the evidence that supports the answer requires us to summarize the key lesson(s) from an episode of evidence-based learning. Writing a concise summary exercises and disciplines our ability to distill the gist of that learning episode, to *consolidate* our learning, helping us get the most out of it.[33] Second, since many important questions are about common disorders and their management, we can expect to need the knowledge more than once. By storing a CAT and retrieving it later, we can make our learning efforts *cumulative* (we start from where we left off last time) rather than *duplicative* (we start all over again). Third, by sharing CATs

---

Table 9.5 Writing structured summaries of evidence-based learning, or critically appraised topics (CATs)

Why use written summaries or CATs?
1. To summarize and consolidate our learning
2. To make our learning cumulative, not duplicative
3. To share our learning efforts with others on our team
4. To refine our EBM skills.

How should we structure evidence summaries or CATs?
Title: declarative sentence that states the clinical bottom line
Clinical Question: 4 (or 3) components of the foreground question that started it all
Clinical bottom line: concise statement of best available answer(s) to the question
Evidence summary: description of methods and/or results in concise form (e.g., table)
Comments: about evidence (e.g., limitations) or how to use it in your own setting
Citation(s): include evidence appraised and other resources, if appropriate
Appraiser: so you'll know who did the appraising when you return to it later
Date CAT was "born"/expiration date: so folks will know when to look again.

9

with others on our clinical team, they can learn from our efforts, too, so learning can multiply. Keep in mind that CATs are most useful to those who make them. Fourth, with repetition and coaching, writing CATs can help us refine our EBM skills.

Incorporating EBM into existing educational sessions

In the foregoing discussion, we've emphasized strategies and tactics for individual clinical teachers who want to add evidence to the mix of what they teach, whether in Modes 1, 2 or 3. Some of us have the added responsibility of planning how to introduce EBM into existing educational sessions and conferences, so we address here some of the considerations in doing this, illustrating with two common states, "Morning Report" and "Journal Club".

Morning Report

In many centers, the individual team's post-call rounds are supplemented by a service-wide conference called Morning Report. We've witnessed more than 60 variations of this conference in our travels, although most share six characteristics: most of the senior residents on the clinical service are present, including chief resident(s); faculty who attend often include the program director and/or departmental chair; one (or a few) recent admission(s) are presented, although they vary in newness; the cases are selected for their potential educational value; the discussions vary widely, but usually focus on the initial diagnosis and treatment of the presented patients' conditions; and, follow-up on prior discussed cases can be presented, with occasional educational extras.[34]

The Morning Report has several features that make it uniquely attractive as a place to start integrating EBM into the program's curriculum. Clinical learners present real patients with real illnesses, and discuss real clinical decisions that need to be made in real-time. If a safe and stimulating learning climate has been established, learners can identify what they do and don't know yet in order to make these decisions wisely, yielding many questions that could be asked. Because Morning Report occurs repeatedly, its multiple sessions allow learning to be multi-staged. Also, as evidence and other knowledge are learned and shared among those who attend, the judgments involved in integrating and applying the new knowledge can be explicitly addressed. Given the high visibility of the conference, particularly when it's actively supported by the departmental leadership, learners can see the importance placed on learning clinical medicine in evidence-based ways and the development of lifelong learning skills. Comparing these features to the above list of 10 successes in teaching EBM shows how much potential success Morning Report could have.

Yet Morning Report may also present you with several challenges to incorporating EBM. First, if those who run Morning Report have other goals for the session, such as using the time for record-keeping duties, these competing objectives can consume learning time, destroy the learning climate or derail the learning process altogether. Second, if cases are not presented concisely, so much time can be spent sorting through the clinical data that little time is left for learning, including learning how to inform decisions with evidence. Third, if the learning climate is unsafe, or if learners' ability to ask questions is reduced, then few of the learners' actual knowledge gaps may get asked as questions. Fourth, teacher or learner inexperience with EBM may lead some participants to retreat to pathophysiologic rationale or personal experience when deciding between test or treatment strategies, rather than risk exposing their rudimentary EBM skills by considering evidence to inform their decisions. Specifically, poor question formulation may lead the group's learning astray, while poor searching may frustrate attempts to find current best evidence, and poor critical appraisal skills may lead to the unwise use of flawed evidence in decisions. Fifth, in some centers, those who attend Morning Report change very frequently, which confounds attempts to make learning multi-staged, and might require repeated re-orientation to how to use EBM in Morning Report, as skills can drift between rotations.

Despite these challenges, our own and others' experiences suggest that Morning Report can become a popular and enduring conference in which to incorporate EBM.[35,36] Although occasionally we might model evidence-based practice, in Mode 1, Morning Report is well suited mostly for weaving evidence into teaching clinical medicine (Mode 2), and for targeted teaching of EBM skills (Mode 3). Reflecting on how we've taught in Mode 3 during Morning Report, we find that we emphasize some skills (such as asking questions and integrating the evidence with other knowledge into decisions), while mentioning but not emphasizing other skills (such as searching or critical appraisal), as outlined in Table 9.6. Others we've seen put different emphasis on various EBM skills, sometimes devoting whole sessions of Morning Report to searching or critical appraisal.

To help you prepare to successfully introduce EBM into your Morning Report, we suggest these six maneuvers. First, find and cultivate allies

9

Table 9.6 Developing EBM skills in and out of Morning Report		
EBM skill	**During Morning Report**	**Elsewhere**
Asking questions	In context: cases, decisions Model and see modeled Question drills Practice and feedback.	Read materials on how to ask answerable questions Attend how-to sessions; 1-on-1 coaching See modeled elsewhere.
Searching for evidence	Review searches briefly Explain options briefly Invite clinical librarian Refine, not learn anew.	Read about searching Attend how-to sessions 1-on-1 coaching See modeled elsewhere.
Critical appraisal	Discuss appraisal briefly Teaching scripts about selected portions Refine, not learn anew.	Read about appraisal Attend how-to sessions 1-on-1 coaching See modeled elsewhere.
Integration into decisions	In context: cases, decisions Make judgments explicit Integrate values explicitly Identify factors to weigh.	Read about integration Attend how-to sessions 1-on-1 coaching See modeled elsewhere.
Self evaluation	Model, esp. at beginning Use checklists Increase reflection, self-awareness, insight Group feedback.	Read about self-evaluation Attend how-to sessions 1-on-1 coaching See modeled elsewhere.

who will work with you and advocate for an evidence-based approach to learning in Morning Report. Some may be in your program, such as chief residents and faculty, while others may be in other disciplines, including librarians, statisticians, and clinical pharmacists. Second, negotiate teaching and learning EBM to be part of the goals and methods of Morning Report, by meeting with or becoming the folks who run the conference at your institution. This may take repeated efforts at persuasion, so be persistent. Third, if possible, simultaneously negotiate the use of group learning techniques and the development of a healthy learning climate into your Morning Report, since they are both so important to success.[37] Fourth, help assemble the infrastructure needed to learn, practice and teach in evidence-based ways, including quick access to evidence resources and opportunities to learn more about EBM skills outside of Morning Report. Fifth, prepare some learning materials for EBM, including introductory materials on how to get started, samples of concise evidence summaries, whether your own CATs or from evidence-based pre-appraised sources, and concise explanations of methods underlying the practice of EBM. Sixth, refine further your own skills in facilitating group discussions and in teaching EBM, whether by getting local coaching or by attending a course in how to teach EBM.

On the first day, use most of that Morning Report session to get the group off to a great start, using six tactics. First, identify the main learning goals for your Morning Report and how EBM fits in – ours are "to improve our abilities to think through our cases with explicit clinical reasoning and to learn from our cases with evidence-based medicine." Second, have participants assess their current skills for each main learning goal, both globally and for each skill. Try the "double you" format: "How comfortable do *you* feel with *your* ability to … ?" Don't forget to celebrate learners' courage when they acknowledge they need help. Third, have participants set specific goals for learning EBM in Morning Report, taking care to help them set specific goals that are realistic and focused on their own learning needs. Fourth, negotiate the specific formats you'll use to achieve those learning goals, including issues about the case discussions (e.g., How detailed should presentations be? How focused should the discussion be?), about the EBM portions (e.g., How many questions should we aim to formulate? How often should each learner present an Educational Prescription?), and about how much time you'll spend on each. Fifth, negotiate the ground rules for the group's learning efforts in Morning Report, including both general issues and any specific to the use of evidence (see suggestions in Table 9.9). Sixth, plan when in the rotation you'll revisit the group's learning objectives and adjust the group's methods – we usually do it both at mid-cycle and at the end of the rotation.

Once your Morning Report is up and running, using a combination of case discussions and Educational Prescriptions (Ch. 1), you may find the following six tactics useful. First, during the case presentations, listen "with both ears" to diagnose both the case and the learner, staying alert to both verbal and non-verbal cues. We use a list of common types of clinical questions (Ch. 1) to help us spot clinical issues and learning needs. Second, help the group select one or a few issues of the case to discuss well, rather than aiming to cover the entire case superficially. This allows the group to pool its knowledge, and find its knowledge gaps, on the way to making sound and explicitly informed decisions. Third, help learners articulate these knowledge gaps as answerable clinical questions, and guide them explicitly in the selection of which questions to pursue. Fourth, as learners report their Educational Prescriptions, listen carefully to select one (or a very few) teaching point(s) to make

9

about applying this evidence for the decision at hand. Fifth, if needed, be ready to provide a brief (2–5 min) explanation of one aspect of critical appraisal that has special bearing on the evidence at hand, referring those interested in learning more to sources outside of Morning Report. Sixth, when debriefing the chief residents after Morning Report about their teaching skills, include teaching EBM along with the other topics in your coaching.

Journal Club

In many clinical centers, Journal Clubs run like Cheyne–Stokes breathing, alternating a few raspy grunts with prolonged apneic inactivity. Many seem to confuse newness with importance, so on a rotating schedule, the participants are asked to summarize the latest issues of pre-assigned journals. This means that the choice of topics is driven not by patients' or learners' needs, but instead either by the investors, investigators and editors who choose which products get studied and which get published, or by the postal workers and web servers who determine which journals get delivered. Little wonder, then, that so many learners find their Journal Clubs to be so suffocating.

Yet some Journal Clubs are flourishing,[38] and a growing number of them are designed and conducted along EBM lines.[39-43] In the many variations we've run, seen or read about, three different learning goals can be identified: learning about the best evidence to inform clinical decisions, learning about important new evidence that should change our practice, or building EBM skills. While Journal Clubs can have more than one learning goal, several of the curricular choices made will depend on which goal is pre-eminent (Table 9.7). Although departments will vary in the choices they make, many will recognize that taking the "skills driven" approach first will lead to greater subsequent success with either the "needs driven" or "evidence driven" versions.

To help you prepare to successfully introduce EBM into your Journal Club, we suggest these six maneuvers. First, find and cultivate the allies, whether from in your department or elsewhere, who will help you achieve your aims. Second, negotiate teaching and learning EBM to be one of the main goals of Journal Club, either by meeting with or by becoming those who run the conference. While you're at it, try to negotiate departmental consensus on which of the three learning goals in Table 9.7 will be pre-eminent at your institution. Third, negotiate the use of group learning techniques and the development of a healthy learning climate into your Journal Club. Fourth, help assemble the infrastructure needed to learn, practice and teach in evidence-based

Table 9.7 Three (potentially competing) goals for evidence-based Journal Clubs

	Needs driven	Evidence driven	Skills driven
What is the main learning goal?	Learn how best to handle patient problems that are common, serious or vexing.	Learn about advances in medical knowledge that should change our practice.	Learn the skills for evidence-based practice.
What group learning needs are identified?	Group members identify what patient problems they need most help with.	Group members identify in what aspects or field they aim to keep current.	Group members identify what skills for evidence-based practice they need most to refine.
What type of evidence is valued most?	Current best evidence useful for solving problems, of several types (see Table 1.2), even if not brand new or not strong.	Recent advances in the field that are valid, important and applicable enough to change our practice (i.e., both new and strong).	Evidence that best allows learners to develop the skills they need, of broad range of types (see Table 1.2), even if not brand new or not strong.
Who should select topics and types of evidence?	All participants who share responsibility for solving patient problems.	All participants who share responsibility for staying current.	Members (usually faculty) responsible for finding learning needs and helping learners develop their skills.
Which EBM teaching mode is pre-eminent?	Mode 2 (learning good clinical practice in evidence-based ways).	Mode 2 (developing current awareness in evidence-based ways).	Mode 3 (learning EBM skills).

9

ways, including quick access to evidence resources and opportunities to learn more about EBM skills outside of Journal Club. Fifth, prepare some learning materials for EBM, including introductory materials on how to get started, samples of concise evidence summaries, whether your own CATs or from evidence-based pre-appraised sources, and even concise explanations of methods underlying the practice of EBM. Sixth, refine further your own skills in facilitating group discussions and in teaching EBM, whether by getting local coaching or by attending a course in how to teach EBM.

No matter how the learning goals in Table 9.7 are balanced, we've noticed that most evidence-based Journal Clubs appear to be based on either a three-session cycle or a two-session cycle. In the three-session model, each Journal Club session can be thought of as consisting of three parts.

In Part 1, Journal Club members identify some learning needs to be addressed in the future. For a "needs driven" group, this can take the form of learners presenting cases where they faced uncertainty in clinical decisions, continuing until there is group consensus that a particular problem is worth the time and effort necessary to find its solution. For an "evidence driven" group, group members can debate which part of their field they most need to update. For a "skills driven" group, the members would discuss and decide which skill for evidence-based practice they most need to develop or refine. No matter which of these three approaches is taken, the group poses one or more answerable clinical questions (usually foreground ones, as in Ch. 1) with which to start the evidence-based learning episode. Group members take responsibility (either volunteering or on rotation) for performing a search for evidence to be used – whether the best available for the problem, the newest strong evidence for the field segment, or a useful teaching example for the skill. Groups may have members do this in pairs or triplets, so more experienced members can teach skills to newer recruits.

In Part 2, the results of the evidence search on the previous session's problem, field segment, or skill are shared in the form of photocopies of the abstracts of 4–6 systematic reviews, original articles or other evidence. Club members decide which one or two pieces of evidence are worth studying and arrangements are made to get copies of the clinical question and evidence to all members well in advance of the next meeting.

Part 3 is the main part of the Journal Club, and it comprises the critical appraisal of the evidence found in response to a clinical question posed two sessions ago and selected for detailed study last session. This segment often begins with the admission that most learners haven't read the articles, so time (6–10 min) can be provided for everyone to see if they can determine the validity and clinical applicability of one of the articles, reinforcing rapid critical appraisal. After that interlude, the evidence is critically appraised for its validity, importance and applicability and a decision is made about whether and how it could be applied to the patient problems (for "needs driven" groups), whether and how it should change current practice (for "evidence driven" groups), or whether and how it can build skills for evidence-based practice (for "skills driven" groups). Since this is the "pay-off" part of Journal Club, members may need to be guided to complete Parts 1 and 2, so there's time for Part 3. The order of these three parts of Journal Club could be reversed, depending on local preferences.

Alternatively, evidence-based Journal Clubs can be built on a two-session cycle, with only two of the three elements, question development and evidence appraisal.[41] This omits the consideration of and selection from the search output, which may fit learners who have already mastered searching and selecting. The two-session cycle allows more questions to be addressed over 1 year's calendar, without increasing the duration of each session.

These two conferences, Morning Report and Journal Club, illustrate many of the considerations involved when reorienting existing conferences along evidence-based lines. In more general and explicit form, we've gathered, in Table 9.8, our favorite 20 questions to ask when integrating EBM into a conference, grouped into issues of persons, places, times, things, and ideas.

Integrating EBM into a curriculum

Some of us are also responsible for introducing EBM into the curricula of either undergraduate or graduate medical educational programs.[44-46] For those who want to learn more about curricula in general and how to develop, implement and evaluate them, we refer you to other works on these topics.[47-52]

Learners need to learn not only how to practice each EBM step, but also when to do each step and how to integrate EBM with the other tasks of clinical work. In this way, learning EBM resembles learning other complex "clinical process" skills like the medical interview and the physical examination. To learn such complex undertakings requires not only beginning with a good introduction, but also revisiting the field numerous times building on those experiences that came before. This learning trajectory describes an ascending and outwardly curving spiral, allowing each return to subjects to be vertically aligned with prior teaching.

247

Table 9.8 20 questions for integrating EBM into a learning session

Persons:
1. Who will be the learners, and what are their learning abilities and needs?
2. Who will be the teachers, and what are their teaching strengths and passions?
3. Who will need to serve as allies or permission-givers for this to succeed?
4. What conversations and relationships need to be developed for this to succeed?

Places:
5. Where will this learning session be held?
6. How might the physical space help or hinder learning?
7. How can the physical space be altered to optimize learning?

Times:
8. When and for how long will this learning session be held?
9. Can the sessions be scheduled to support multiple learning stages?
10. How much time will teachers and learners need to prepare for this session?
11. How much time will learners need after this session to receive feedback and to reflect upon, consolidate, clarify, and extend their learning?
12. How much time will teachers need after this session to give feedback and to reflect upon, cultivate and refine their teaching?

Things:
13. What resources need to be present during the learning session?
14. What resources need to be available for teachers and learners before and after the session?
15. How should participants summarize their evidence-based learning, e.g., CATs or Educational Prescriptions?
16. What tools of measurement, assessment, and evaluation will be used for this session?

Ideas:
17. How well does EBM fit with the other goals of this learning session?
18. How can the learning climate be optimized for an evidence-based approach?
19. Which modes of teaching EBM should be emphasized in this session?
20. How many of the 10 features of success in teaching EBM can be included; how many of the 10 mistakes in teaching EBM can be avoided?

How can we start building this vertically aligned spiral trajectory that integrates EBM into a curriculum? We'll illustrate our suggestions using the 4-year undergraduate medical curriculum template found in many North American medical schools. Since Flexner's time, these 4 years have usually comprised 2 years of pre-clinical study separate from 2 years of clinical rotations.[53]

As you build or revise your curriculum, we suggest attention to nine of its general aspects that can improve the fit of EBM at your institution. First, establish the overall learning goals you want students to achieve and competencies you want students to demonstrate by graduation. For instance, many schools have examined the Accreditation Council for Graduate Medical Education's six core competencies for graduate medical education – medical knowledge, patient care, communication, professionalism, systems-based practice, and practice-based learning and improvement – and are adopting and adapting these for use with undergraduate learners. Doing so creates some sensible "homes" for student competence in EBM and lifelong learning, as it connects to several of the core competencies, particularly with practice-based learning and improvement. Second, rather than have students study for separate, discipline-based courses, build the curriculum so students learn the biologic sciences, the clinical sciences, and the social sciences relevant to medicine in a fully integrated way.[54,55] Doing so provides them with deliberate practice in integrating the evidence from clinical care research with other knowledge to inform their decisions. Third, identify authentic healthcare contexts (across the spectrum of care) for the content students are expected to learn, organized around the decisions to make, problems to solve, conversations to hold and actions to carry out that will be expected of them upon graduation. Doing this helps students find motivation to learn, helps students and teachers select what is relevant to learn, and provides a concrete situation to apply what is learned.[19] This parallels the "real patients, real decisions" advice we mentioned earlier for individual teachers. Fourth, plan how and where in the curriculum to address all four domains of learning: affective, cognitive, conative, and psychomotor.[21] Doing so helps students develop well-rounded skills for clinical practice, into which EBM and lifelong learning can easily fit. Fifth, plan purposefully how you will balance passive learning strategies such as assigned reading or web modules, with active learning strategies, such as problem-based learning,[56-62] team-based learning[63,64] or other active methods.[18,19,65] Doing so will ensure that students will have many opportunities to engage with problems or decisions, discover their knowledge gaps and learning needs, and then get coached on asking questions, finding answers, appraising the answers, applying answers to the problem under study, and deciding how to act. Sixth, since these motivated and curious students will want to learn a great deal, it follows they will need a rich array of learning resources assembled to help them, including not only knowledge collections such as the medical literature and multi-media learning resources,[66,67] but also extensive simulation and skill-building resources.[68-71] Seventh, since these engaged learners will want to know how they are progressing in developing competence, and since schools and society will be holding students accountable for learning, a robust

9

program of assessments should be planned in the curriculum that aligns both formative and summative assessments with the learning objectives, activities, and so forth.[21],[72–75] Doing so creates the context into which assessments of EBM and lifelong learning skills would readily fit. Eighth, recruit, cultivate, and maintain a critical mass of excellent educators,[76,77] who can teach in the several different roles needed by students in this type of curriculum.[21] Doing so should maximize the students' exposure to excellent role models who teach EBM in all three modes. Ninth, establish a healthy learning climate that balances a high degree of intellectual challenge and engagement with a high degree of personal support and interpersonal collaboration. Doing so won't eliminate students' cognitive dissonance when they encounter the need to learn more, but it can help them respond to this dissonance in adaptive and constructive fashion.

With these general curricular issues addressed, you can turn to six aspects specific to EBM and lifelong learning. First, find and cultivate allies who will work with you and advocate for an evidence-based approach to learning throughout the curriculum. Some of these allies may already be in your school, including other faculty, residents, librarians, and others. Others may be closer than you think, such as in nearby colleges of public health or pharmacy. Second, negotiate that learning EBM becomes an important theme of your curriculum, and this too may take persistence. Our experience suggest that this often means you have to become the person or team that builds and runs this theme, so be prepared. Third, adopt an overall curricular schema of EBM to use in planning and sequencing. We include in Figure 9.1 the one we use. This three dimensional grid shows on

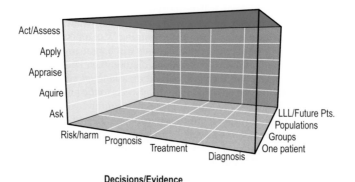

Decisions/Evidence

Figure 9.1 A curricular grid for EBM in medical education.

its *x* axis the four main categories of clinical decisions (as in four chapters in this book): Risk or Harm, Prognosis, Treatment, and Diagnosis; on its *y* axis the five main skills dealt with in the other chapters in this book: Asking questions, Acquiring the evidence, Appraising evidence critically, Applying or integrating into clinical decisions, and Assessing the process and impact of acting on the evidence; and on its *z* axis, the healthcare context in which these decisions are being made (for individual patients, for groups of patients, for whole populations, or for future patients). Fourth, using this grid, select milestones for each box in the grid that build toward competence and are developmentally appropriate for each stage of the curriculum. For instance, we think that students should be able to ask answerable questions and search for evidence independently by the time they arrive on their clinical rotations. Fifth, create curricular modules with detailed learning objectives, learning activities, learning resources, and assessment strategies to help students achieve these developmental milestones at the appropriate times. Sixth, embed these curricular modules into the 4-year calendar, and integrate into the relevant workflow, syllabi, and examinations.

How might such a curriculum look? Although they may not yet be directly responsible for the care of patients, students in the first 2 years can nonetheless look ahead and engage with realistic clinical or population health situations. For instance, even on the first day of school, students have heard that smoking increases the risk of various diseases, or that influenza vaccines are recommended annually for many population subgroups. Thus, as the principles of EBM are introduced to them in Mode 3 and they encounter the four decision types of the *x* axis and the five skills of the *y* axis, students can be actively engaged in addressing authentic healthcare contexts. Because some of the skills of EBM take time to practice before use in direct patient care, we and others have chosen to introduce the principles of EBM in the first and second pre-clerkship years.[55,78] Several learning approaches can be combined, including interactive large groups and team-based learning, along with small-group and self-directed learning sessions to help students build their fundamental skills on the *y* axis for the main four decision types on the *x* axis, with a representative sample of healthcare contexts on the *z* axis. Throughout the entire pre-clerkship curriculum, students could encounter teachers who teach in Modes 1 and 2.

Once in their clinical rotations during years 3 and 4, we expect students to be exposed to the opposite proportions of teaching modes: theoretically nearly every clinician could role model EBM practice and weave evidence into their clinical teaching, while fewer opportunities may

9

be available to teach the fundamental EBM skills. Students who have had a sound introduction to the principles and skills during the first 2 years could be asked to practice these skills deliberately, such as by writing and presenting CATs on each clinical team they join, and by taking part in the departmental Morning Reports and Journal Clubs, as described above. During elective periods, such as in the final 4th year, students could have the option of taking an advanced course in EBM. Over the period of two decades that we've run these advanced EBM electives for selected learners, we have found the grid in Figure 9.1 has helped our students identify the advanced topics they want to learn more about, so that we can tailor the elective toward their learning needs.

Learning more about how to teach EBM

As with any complex craft that's built on experience as well as knowledge, becoming excellent at teaching EBM requires extensive deliberate practice.[11] In addition to trying out the strategies and tactics in this chapter, we suggest five additional ideas. First, keep a teaching journal, in which you record your observations and interpretations of which teaching methods you've tried, what specifically worked, what specifically you'd like to do better, and what you find in watching others teach and in reading about teaching and learning.[79] Second, look for excellent teachers in your institution who would be willing to observe your teaching and provide individualized feedback and coaching, then work with these mentors to develop your skills. Some institutions have formal teaching consultation services available to observe teachers and provide feedback.[80] Third, track down the published series of EBM teaching tips that tackle how to handle teaching difficult material,[81-91] and try using them in your own teaching practice. Don't forget to record your observations and reflections in your teaching journal. Fourth, attend one of the growing number of workshops on "How to teach EBM" being held around the world, which provide you with time for deliberate practice and the opportunity to gain useful feedback on your teaching methods. Fifth, because learning in small groups is so much a part of clinical learning and teaching, and because when group learning works well it can powerfully enhance evidence-based learning, we suggest you devote substantial time and effort to refining your skills for learning and teaching in small groups, starting with the material in Table 9.9 and continuing with additional readings.[92-99] Although connected to teaching, the self-evaluation of learning, practicing and teaching EBM is so important that it deserves its own chapter, (Chapter 8).

Table 9.9 Tips for teaching EBM in clinical teams and other small groups[a]

Help team/group members understand why to learn in small groups

Learners may vary in their prior experiences with learning in groups, so they may benefit from reflecting on why it's worth undertaking. Useful points are:

1. Learning in groups allows a broader range of questions about any given topic to be asked and answered, since the work is done by several people. As the results of an individual's effort are shared with others, lessons learned have a "multiplier" effect.
2. Learning in groups allows experienced members to pair with inexperienced members during the work, thereby helping novices to learn faster and reinforcing everyone's capacity for teamwork.
3. The interactive discussions groups use as they learn can help individual members clarify their own misconceptions, consolidate the lessons learned by explaining things to others, and hear multiple viewpoints when considering the implications of the new knowledge for decision and action.
4. Learning in groups allows individual participants to practice performance of skills, using other group members within practice, which helps the individual to learn.
5. Learning in groups also allows individual participants to get feedback on their performance from peers as well as tutors, providing both a "reality check" to their own perceptions and suggestions for further learning.
6. The camaraderie, the interpersonal support, and the cohesion from shared challenges and achievements can make learning in groups more fun than learning in isolation.
7. In many fields of work, leaders spend time building groups of individuals into well-functioning work teams, since team performance almost always bests that of individuals.
8. Consider an analogy between group learning and how professional cyclists ride in groups – by riding closely in the peloton to draft and to rotate leading, cyclists can ride faster, longer and farther than even the best of them can ride individually.

Help team/group members set sensible ground rules for small group learning

Small groups can succeed in learning EBM (or anything else) if group members establish effective ways of working together. Useful ground rules include the following:

1. Members take responsibility (individually and as a group) for:
   a. Showing up, and on time
   b. Learning each other's names, interests and objectives
   c. Respecting each other
   d. Removing distractions, such as audible tones, games, or communications on mobile phones and computers
   e. Contributing to, accepting, and supporting individual and group rules of behavior, including confidentiality
   f. Contributing to, accepting, and supporting both the overall objectives of the group and the detailed plans and assignments for each session
   g. Carrying out the agreed-upon plans and assignments, including role-playing
   h. Listening (concentrating and analyzing), rather than simply preparing your own response to what's being said
   i. Talking (including consolidating and summarizing).

(Continued)

9

Table 9.9 Tips for teaching EBM in clinical teams and other small groups[a]—Cont'd

2. Members monitor and (by using time in/time out) reinforce positive and correct negative elements of both:
   a. "Process", including:
      - Educational methods, e.g., reinforcing positive contributions and teaching methods; proposing strategies for improving less effective ones
      - Group functioning, e.g., identifying behaviors, not motives; encouraging non-participants; quieting down over-participators.
   b. "Content", including:
      - Critical appraisal topics, e.g., if unclear, uncertain or incorrect facts or principles, strategies, or tactics about how to carry it out
      - Clinical matters, e.g., if clinical context or usefulness is unclear.
3. Members evaluate self, each other, the group, the session, and the program with candor and respect:
   a. Celebrating what went well and what should be preserved
   b. Identifying what went less well, focusing on strategies for correcting or improving the situation.
4. When giving feedback constructively, members do the following:
   a. Give feedback only when asked to do so or when the offer is accepted
   b. Give feedback as soon after the event as possible
   c. Focus on the positive; wherever possible give positive feedback first and last
   d. Be descriptive (of behavior), not evaluative (of motives)
   e. Talk about specific behaviors and give examples where possible
   f. Use "I" and give your experience of the behavior
   g. When giving negative feedback, suggest alternative behaviors
   h. Confine negative feedback to behaviors that can be changed
   i. Ask, "Why am I giving this feedback?" (Is it really to help the person concerned?)
   j. Remember that feedback says a lot about its giver as well as its receiver.
5. When receiving feedback constructively, members do the following:
   a. Listen to it (rather than prepare a response or defense)
   b. Ask for it to be repeated if it wasn't easily heard
   c. Ask for clarification and examples if statements are unclear or unsupported
   d. Assume it is constructive until proven otherwise; then, use and consider those elements that are constructive
   e. Pause and think before responding
   f. Accept it positively (for consideration) rather than dismissively (for self-protection)
   g. Ask for suggestions of specific ways to modify or change the behavior
   h. Respect and thank the person giving feedback.

Help team/group members plan the learning activities wisely

During initial introductions, group members should identify their individual learning goals, from which the group can set group learning goals. Tutors and group members should keep these learning goals in mind as they plan the learning objectives for each session, including what to learn, what to emphasize, and how to engage the group in the learning activities. For groups just beginning to learn EBM, consider the following:

Table 9.9 Tips for teaching EBM in clinical teams and other small groups[a]—Cont'd

1. Plan the session to include a learning situation that is realistic to what group members do in their actual work. For most clinicians, this means using the illnesses of patients actually in their care, or case examples they might encounter frequently.
2. Prepare the question, search and critical appraisal ahead of time, to be familiar with the teaching challenges that may arise. Of the possible questions this case could generate, select one with a high yield in terms of learning, which is usually a mix of the following considerations:
   a. Relevance to the clinical decision being made
   b. Appropriateness to the learners' prior knowledge
   c. Availability of good-quality evidence to address the question (so first experience shows positively how evidence can be used once understood and appraised)
   d. Availability of easily understood evidence about the question (so first experience is not too overwhelming methodologically)
   e. Likelihood the question will recur, so learners can benefit more than once.
3. As the session begins, engage the group in the clinical situation and have the group focus on the decision to be made. Consider having group members vote on what they would do clinically before the evidence is appraised (if need be, this can be done anonymously).
4. Encourage group members to run the session, yet be prepared to guide them in the early going.
5. As the group works through the critical appraisal portions, emphasize how to understand and use research, rather than how to do research.
6. Summarize important points in the session (if the group is using a scribe, this person could record them for later retrieval).
7. As the session ends, encourage the group to come to closure on how to use the evidence in the clinical decision. Keep in mind that coming to closure needn't require complete agreement; rather, a good airing of the issues that ends in legitimate disagreement can be very instructive.
8. Keep to the time plan overall, but don't worry if the group doesn't cover everything in this one session – if the initial experience goes well, there will be more opportunities.
9. For groups gaining competence and confidence in EBM, the sky is the limit. Encourage the group to invent its own activities, and consider the following:
   a. When selecting questions and evidence to appraise, consider using:
      • Flawed evidence, so the group can develop skill in detecting flaws
      • A pair of articles, one good and one not so good, for the group to compare
      • A pair of good articles that reach opposite conclusions
      • Controversial evidence, so the group learns to disagree constructively
      • Evidence that debunks current practice, so the group learns to question carefully
      • A systematic review of early small trials, along with a later definitive trial.
   b. When selecting learning contexts to employ in the group, encourage group members to try out sessions of increasing difficulty, such as practicing teaching jaded senior residents or registrars rather than eager students.

9

(Continued)

Table 9.9 Tips for teaching EBM in clinical teams and other small groups[a]—Cont'd

c. When group members disagree, capitalize on the disagreement, by such tactics as:
- Trying to sort out whether the disagreement is about the data, the critical appraisal, or the values we use in making the judgments
- Framing the disagreement positively, as a chance to understand more deeply
- Framing the protagonists positively, as providing the group a chance to learn by stating the various perspectives on the topic
- Wherever possible, keeping the disagreement from becoming personal, and avoiding trying to defend the article.

Help team/group members keep a healthy learning climate

The learning climate is the general tone and atmosphere that pervades the group sessions. Encourage the group to cultivate a safe, positive learning climate, wherein group members feel comfortable identifying their limitations and addressing them. Some tactics include the following:

1. Be honest and open about your own limitations and the things you don't know.
2. Model the behavior of turning what you don't know into answerable questions and following through on finding answers, using an educational prescription.
3. Have fun with, and show others the fun in, finding knowledge gaps and learning.
4. Encourage all questions, particularly those that aim for deep understanding.
5. Encourage legitimate disagreement, particularly when handled constructively.
6. Encourage group members to use educational prescriptions.
7. Provide both intellectual challenge (to stimulate learning) and personal support (to help make learning adaptive).

Help team/group members keep the discussion going

1. Early on, model effective facilitating behaviors that encourage discussion, such as:
   a. When someone asks a question, turn the question over to the group and ask them
   b. If a group member answers another member's question well, ask others in the group for additional effective ways that they've used to answer the same question
   c. If a group discussion turns into a debate between two members, ask others to provide additional perspective before the group decides
   d. Don't be afraid of quiet moments, and of using silence when needed.
2. Observe carefully how group members keep discussion moving, and use these observations for feedback and coaching.
3. Encourage group members to reflect on what works well in different teaching situations, and provide each other feedback on this, balancing the desire to move forward with the need to pull everyone along.

Table 9.9 Tips for teaching EBM in clinical teams and other small groups[a]—Cont'd

Help team/group members keep the discussion on track

1. Early on, model effective facilitating behaviors that help group members to stay focused on the task at hand, such as:
   a. Break the discussion into observable chunks, and set short time for each chunk, e.g., "For the next 2 min, let's brainstorm all the outcomes of clinical interest to us for this condition and its treatment"
   b. When someone brings up a tangent, identify it non-judgmentally and ask the group how they'd like to handle it
   c. Reflect to the group what they seem to be discussing, to inform their choices about how to spend their efforts.
2. Observe carefully how group members keep the discussion on track, and use these observations for feedback and coaching.
3. Encourage group members to reflect on what works well for keeping a discussion focused well, while at the same time staying alert for good teaching moments that arise spontaneously.

Help team/group members manage time well

To accomplish their group objectives, group members need to manage their time together effectively. This includes spending time on things that are important and avoiding distractions wherever possible. Some tactics include:

1. At the beginning, model effective time management by encouraging the group to set specific plans for how much time to spend on:
   a. Carrying out the learning activities for the present session
   b. Evaluating the present session, including giving feedback
   c. Planning the subsequent session, including revising group objectives.
2. As the group takes charge, coach the members on issues of time management, such as:
   a. How to use a "timekeeper", usually a member not leading that session
   b. How to adjust time allotted for various functions, after group negotiation
   c. How to handle new learning issues that arise, which might consume time to address. Here several options exist, including the following:
      • Address it fully right then (if it's important enough and if the group's work would halt without doing so)
      • Address it briefly at the time, and have a group member (or tutor) address it more completely later, either to the group or with the individual
      • Delay addressing the topic; instead, record it for later discussion (in a place sometimes dubbed the "parking lot").
3. Encourage the group to evaluate time management as the members evaluate the group's functioning.

Help team/group members address some common issues of learning EBM

Jargon

Jargon consists of words from the technical languages of any discipline; for EBM these can be from epidemiology, biostatistics, decision sciences, economics, and other fields. If unexplained, jargon can be intimidating and might delay learning. Some tactics for dealing with jargon include:

(Continued)

Table 9.9 Tips for teaching EBM in clinical teams and other small groups[a]—Cont'd

1. Introduce and explain the idea first, then label it with the technical term. In this way the understanding comes first, before the word can intimidate.
2. If group members introduce jargon terms, ask them to explain the terms to others in concise ways. This helps the group's understanding, and allows the member to practice brief explanations for later use.
3. Consider having the group keep an accumulating glossary of terms covered, for members to refer to during and after the sessions. You can start with the brief glossary that is in this book (see the Appendix).

Quantitative study results

Most reports contain simple calculations, and many contain complex and intimidating ones. Although most of them don't deserve extensive discussion, others, if left unexplained, can needlessly intimidate some learners. Tactics for dealing with quantitative results are as follows:

1. Introduce the concept using real data and work slowly through the arithmetic, so learners can follow the calculations.
2. Use the word names for the arithmetical functions, rather than talking in symbols.
3. Calculate a result from the study data, then introduce its name and a general formula. Just as in dealing with jargon, this order helps de-mystify the terms.
4. To check their understanding, allow group members time to practice the arithmetic until they feel comfortable enough to move on.
5. Consider having the group keep an accumulating glossary of quantitative results, including names, formulae and uses, for group members to use during and afterwards (see Appendix).

Statistics

The study's methods and results sections will usually describe the technical devices of statistics used for the research. Some may be familiar to you and your group members, while many may not be. Groups will need to learn how to handle questions about statistics, epidemiology, or any other methodological issue. Some tactics include:

1. Highlight the distinction between statistical and clinical significance, and illustrate with evidence being examined.
2. Assuming the group members want to learn how to understand and use research, rather than do research (worth double-checking now and then), consider advising the group to select a few statistical notions to understand well (e.g., confidence intervals, CIs), and point them to resources that can help them.
3. Ask the group how deeply they'd like to delve into this topic (many will opt for shallow initial treatment, to allow the group's work to continue, followed by resources for deeper learning later). If they choose deeper amounts, and you cannot provide this on the spot, involve them in choosing among the realistic alternatives, including:

Table 9.9 Tips for teaching EBM in clinical teams and other small groups[a]—Cont'd

    a. A single group member (or the tutor, if needed) looks up the statistical measure or test and reports back concisely at a later session

    b. Pairs or small teams from the group find the needed information outside the session, and plan a learning activity around it for a subsequent session

    c. A nearby statistician is persuaded to join the group temporarily to address the topic at a subsequent session.

4. Remind group members that they may face learners with similar questions upon return home. Coach them in developing answers of different lengths and depths, appropriate for different situations:

    a. "One liners" – for when learners want just enough to get back to other work

    b. "One paragraphers" – for when learners want more verbal explanation

    c. "One siders" – one page (or a few) handouts on the topic that might be developed ahead of time, for learners who want a little more depth to read later; this can be coupled with "one citers", i.e., a useful citation for even more depth.

5. As the group members run sessions themselves, observe carefully how they handle statistical, epidemiological or other methodological issues and use these observations in coaching and feedback.

6. Ask the group to assess its handling of methodological topics when they evaluate the session.

7. Consider having the group keep a log of methodological issues covered.

Help team/group members identify and deal with counterproductive behaviors

Nihilism

As learners grow in their ability to detect study flaws, some may go through a period of nihilism ("No study is perfect, so what good is any literature?"). Often this occurs in those who can find bias but who don't yet understand its consequences. This negative imbalance is usually temporary, but it can dampen the spirits of others and impede group function. Some tactics are useful in ameliorating this unease:

1. Select good articles at the start, so that early experiences are positive.

2. When using flawed articles, ask the group if something can be learned, even if the study does not provide a definitive answer.

3. Help group members put the study in its knowledge context – what else is known about this? Although potentially flawed, a study may be the earliest in a given field, when the state of prior knowledge is low. Thus, the study may represent incomplete knowledge, rather than bad knowledge.

4. Help group members ask whether missing information is due to poor study design and execution or due to editorial decisions about publishing space. Some data missing in the report may be available from the authors of the study.

5. Help group members separate minor problems from major design flaws that seriously affect the likely validity of results.

6. Help group members ask a series of questions:

    a. Do the study methods allow the possibility of bias?

    b. If so, how much distortion of the results might this bias cause?

    c. If so, in which direction might this bias distort the results?

7. Help group members identify what they would find in an ideal study that answers the question. Then consider how far from ideal is the available evidence.

9

Table 9.9 Tips for teaching EBM in clinical teams and other small groups[a]—Cont'd

Discussion tangents

Small group work can stimulate learners, bringing forth not only discussion ideas that would keep the group on its learning spiral, but also discussion ideas that could take the group elsewhere (tangents from the spiral). The energy released can be invigorating, yet if every topic were to be discussed, the group would not achieve its objectives. Group members need to learn constructive ways of handling possible discussion tangents, some of which are as follows:

1. Identify to the group that a tangent has arisen, validating it as a possibly productive line of learning.
2. Ask the group to choose how to proceed, based on their overall learning goals rather than just the plan for that session. This may mean following the tangent, as it might meet their goals better, or it may mean placing the tangent on a list of topics to address later (the "parking lot"). Either way, encourage the group to decide, letting them know you'll stick with them on either path.
3. Some tangents can be turned into extended loops of the learning spiral. That is, these topics can be briefly and concisely discussed, enough to inform the original discussion, to which the group then returns. It may help to set a time limit for such a tangent, and have the timekeeper help the group keep to the limit.
4. When they're running the session, observe closely how group members deal with tangents and use these observations for feedback and coaching.
5. Encourage the group to assess its management of tangents during its evaluation.

A dominating over-participator

Some groups may have one or more members whose personality or enthusiasm leads them to contribute a great deal, perhaps to the point of dominating the time and impeding the group's work and the other members' learning. Some tactics for dealing with this include:

1. Use non-verbal signals (eye contact, hand gestures, body position, etc.) to encourage this person to become quieter and others to contribute more.
2. Seat this person next to one of the tutors, which can encourage moderation.
3. After this person contributes again, ask several others to contribute. This may take reminding the over-participator to let others have a fair turn to speak.
4. Take a time-out to address the group's process/progress, perhaps by reviewing the group's ground rules about participation, or by asking the group to identify the over-participation and make adjustments. In doing so, focus on the behavior (amount and nature of speech), rather than on the person or the motivations for the behavior.
5. Consider suggesting the device of a "peace pipe". This can be any object (originally an actual tobacco pipe used at Native American gatherings) that signifies the person holding it has permission to speak. When finished speaking, that person may give the object to someone else or place it on the table for anyone to choose. This can be a fun and instructive exercise to try, through which group members can discover both under- and over-participation, as well as how many of them talk at once.

A quiet non-participator

Some group members are quiet initially, as they "warm-up" to the people and the group's activities. Other members may be quiet longer, either from personal style or for other reasons like language skills. Still others may be quiet due to lack

Table 9.9 Tips for teaching EBM in clinical teams and other small groups[a]—Cont'd

of preparation, for fear of embarrassment or due to lack of engagement. While not always pathologic, quietness can be a signal to individual or group troubles. Groups will need tactics to recognize and address members who contribute little:

1. Be sensitive to reasons for quietness and adjust accordingly. If need be, approach the group member between sessions to find out why.
2. Use non-verbal signals (eye contact, hand gestures, body position, etc.) to encourage this person to contribute more.
3. Seat this person next to one of the tutors, which can encourage participation.
4. Take a time-out to address the group's process/progress, perhaps by reviewing the group's ground rules about participation, or by asking the group to identify the under-participation and make adjustments. In doing so, focus on the behavior (amount and nature of speech), rather than on the person or the motivations for the behavior.
5. Consider pairing the quiet person with another group member for an activity, so they can work together on planning and carrying out this activity. Make sure quiet folks (and all group members) feel more supported as they take on challenges in the group.
6. Consider trying the "peace pipe" (see above). For under-participators, tutors and group members can make it a point to pass it to them, asking them to contribute at least a little before passing it on to others.

Help team/group members prepare for using EBM skills "back home"

As they grow in competence and confidence in their EBM skills, group members will begin to confront how to start or advance their use of EBM in their daily work. For clinicians and teachers, this may mean facing for the first time some of the barriers to incorporating evidence in practice addressed elsewhere in this book. (See also the accompanying CD which includes more on the limitations and misunderstandings of EBM.)You can help them prepare to overcome these barriers with a mix of enthusiasm, realism and practicality. Some tactics include:

1. Encourage each group member to select one or a few places to start introducing EBM, rather than trying to start everywhere at once. Consider having them rank three or more candidate activities for introducing EBM, then discussing in buzz groups the advantages and disadvantages of each.
2. Use the group members' collective experience to brainstorm how to prepare to introduce EBM into a given learning activity. This brainstorming might be usefully organized around five areas: persons, places, times, things, and ideas (see Table 8.8), that would need to be considered when introducing EBM "back home".
3. Since changes involving only a few may be easier than changes involving many, it may be wise to work toward an early success by introducing EBM in a way that doesn't require massive shifts in institutional culture. Indeed, the simplest may be a change that involves the actions of only the group member, at least at first. Once momentum is gained, more challenging tasks can be tackled.
4. Encourage group members to be realistic in setting expectations for what can be accomplished early, yet optimistic about what can be achieved in the long term.

[a]*Thanks again to Martha Gerrity and Valerie Lawrence, who compiled an early version of this list that was published in this book's first edition. Since then, we've kept changing the list as we've gained more experience with small group learning, and because we can't resist the urge to tinker!*

9

References

1. Schon DA. *Educating the reflective practitioner*. San Francisco: Jossey-Bass; 1987.

2. Candy PC. *Self-direction for lifelong learning: A comprehensive guide to theory and practice*. San Francisco: Jossey-Bass; 1991.

3. Neighbour R. *The inner apprentice*. Newbury: Petroc Press; 1996.

4. Davis D, Thomson MA. Continuing medical education as a means of lifelong learning. In: Silagy C, Haines A, eds. *Evidence-based practice in primary care*. London: BMJ Books; 1998.

5. Palmer PJ. *The courage to teach*. San Francisco: Jossey-Bass; 1998.

6. Claxton G. *Wise Up: The challenge of lifelong learning*. New York: Bloomsbury; 1999.

7. Davis DA, O'Brien MA, Freemantle NA, et al. Impact of formal continuing medical education: do conferences, workshops, rounds, and other traditional continuing education activities change physician behavior or health care outcomes? *JAMA*. 1999;282:867–894.

8. Bransford JD, Brown AL, Cocking RR. In: Bransford JD, Brown AL, Cocking RR, eds. *How people learn: Brain, mind, experience, and school*. Washington, DC: National Academy Press; 2000.

9. Brown JS, Duguid P. *The social life of information*. Boston: Harvard Business School Press; 2000.

10. Sawyer RK. *The Cambridge handbook of the learning sciences*. Cambridge: Cambridge University Press; 2006.

11. Ericsson KA, Charness N, Feltovich PJ, et al. *The Cambridge handbook of expertise and expert performance*. Cambridge: Cambridge University Press; 2006.

12. Richardson WS. One, two, three, teach! *Evidence-Based Health Care Newslett*. 1999;19:6–7.

13. Richardson WS. Teaching evidence-based practice on foot. *ACP J Club*. 2005;143:A10–A12.

14. Parkes J, Hyde C, Deeks J, et al. Teaching critical appraisal in health care settings. *Cochrane Database Syst Rev*. 2001;(3) CD001270.

15. Straus SE, Ball C, Balcombe N, et al. Teaching evidence-based medicine skills can change practice in a community hospital. *J Gen Intern Med*. 2005;20:340–343.

16. Pinsky LE, Monson D, Irby DM. How excellent teachers are made: reflecting on success to improve teaching. *Adv Health Sci Ed*. 1998;3:207–215.

17. Dodek PM, Sackett DL, Schechter MT. Systolic and diastolic learning: an analogy to the cardiac cycle. *CMAJ*. 1999;160:1475–1477.

18. Prince MJ. Does active learning work? A review of the research. *J Engr Education*. 2004;93:223–231.

19. Prince MJ, Felder RM. Inductive teaching and learning methods: definitions, comparisons, and research bases. *J Engr Education*. 2006;95:123–138.

20. Hurst JW. The over-lecturing and under-teaching of clinical medicine. *Arch Intern Med*. 2004;164:1605–1608.

21. Reeves TC. How do you know they are learning? The importance of alignment in higher education. *Int J Learning Technology*. 2006;2:294–309.

22. Pinsky LE, Irby DM. If at first you don't succeed: Using failure to improve teaching. *Acad Med*. 1997;72:973–976.

23. LeBlanc VR. The effects of acute stress on performance: implications for health professions education. *Acad Med*. 2009;84(suppl 10): S25–S33.

24. Smith R. Thoughts for new medical students at a new medical school. *BMJ*. 2003;327:1430–1433.

25. Reilly BM. Inconvenient truths about effective clinical teaching. *Lancet*. 2007;370:705–711.

26. Ellis J, Mulligan I, Rowe J, et al. Inpatient general medicine is evidence-based. *Lancet*. 1995;346:407–410.

27. Sackett DL, Straus SE. Finding and applying evidence during clinical rounds: the evidence cart. *JAMA*. 1998;280:1336–1338.

28. Richardson WS, Burdette SD. Practice corner: Taking evidence in hand. *ACP J Club*. 2003;138:A9.

29. Richardson WS. One slice or the whole pie? *Evidence-Based Health Care Newslett*. 2001;21:17–18.

30. Irby DM, Wilkerson L. Teaching when time is limited. *BMJ*. 2008;336:384–387.

31. Sprake C, Cantillon P, Metcalf J, et al. Teaching in an ambulatory care setting. *BMJ*. 2008;337:690–692.

32. Sauve S, Lee HN, Meade MO, et al. The critically appraised topic: a practical approach to learning critical appraisal. *Ann Royal Coll Phys Surg Canada*. 1995;28:396–398.

33. Lloyd FJ, Reyna VF. Clinical gist and medical education: Connecting the dots. *JAMA*. 2009;302:1332–1333.

9

34. Amin Z, Guajardo J, Wisniewski W, et al. Morning report: focus and methods over the past three decades. *Acad Med.* 2000;75(suppl 1):S1–S5.

35. Richardson WS. Teaching evidence-based medicine in morning report. *Clin Epidemiol Newslett.* 1993;13:9.

36. Reilly B, Lemon M. Evidence-based morning report: a popular new format in a large teaching hospital. *Am J Med.* 1997;103:419–426.

37. Stinson L, Pearson D, Lucas B. Developing a learning culture: twelve tips for individuals, teams, and organizations. *Med Teacher.* 2006;28:309–312.

38. Ebbert JO, Montori VM, Schultz HJ. The Journal Club in postgraduate medical education: a systematic review. *Med Teacher.* 2001;23:455–461.

39. Dirschl DR, Tornetta P, Bhandari M. Designing, conducting, and evaluating Journal Clubs in orthopedic surgery. *Clin Ortho Rel Res.* 2003;413:146–157.

40. Forsen JW, Hartman JM, Neely JG. Tutorials in clinical research, part VIII: Creating a Journal Club. *Laryngoscope.* 2003;113:475–483.

41. Phillips RS, Glasziou PP. What makes evidence-based Journal Clubs succeed? *ACP J Club.* 2004;140:A11–A12.

42. Doust J, Del Mar CB, Montgomery BD, et al. EBM Journal Clubs in general practice. *Aust Fam Phys.* 2008;37:54–56.

43. Deenadayalan Y, Grimmer-Somers K, Prior M, et al. How to run an effective Journal Club: A systematic review. *J Eval Clin Pract.* 2008;14(5):898–911.

44. Dawes M, Summerskill W, Glasziou P, et al. Sicily statement of evidence-based practice. *BMC Med Educ.* 2005;5:1.

45. Hatala R, Keitz SA, Wilson MC, et al. Beyond Journal Clubs: Moving toward an integrated evidence-based medicine curriculum. *J Gen Intern Med.* 2006;21:538–541.

46. Glasziou P, Burls A, Gilbert R. Evidence-based medicine and the medical curriculum: The search engine is now as essential as the stethoscope. *BMJ.* 2008;337:704–705.

47. Hunter KM. Eating the curriculum. *Acad Med.* 1997;72(3):167–172.

48. Kern DE, Thomas PA, Howard DM, et al. *Curriculum development for medical education: A six-step approach.* Baltimore: Johns Hopkins University Press; 1998.

49. Ornstein AC, Hunkins FP. In: Ornstein AC, Hunkins FP, eds. *Curriculum: Foundations, principles, and issues.* 3rd ed. Boston: Allyn and Bacon; 1998.

50. Green ML. Identifying, appraising, and implementing medical education curricula: a guide for medical educators. *Ann Intern Med*. 2001;135:889–896.

51. Kaufman DM. ABC of learning and teaching in medicine: Applying educational theory in practice. *BMJ*. 2003;326:213–216.

52. Prideaux D. ABC of learning and teaching in medicine: Curriculum design. *BMJ*. 2003;326:268–270.

53. Fincher RM, Wallach PM, Richardson WS. Basic science right, not basic science lite: Medical education at a crossroad. *J Gen Intern Med*. 2009;24:1255–1258.

54. Neville AJ, Norman GR. PBL in the undergraduate MD program at McMaster University: Three iterations in three decades. *Acad Med*. 2007;82:370–374.

55. Wilkerson L, Stevens CM, Krasne S. No content without context: Integrating basic, clinical, and social sciences in a pre-clerkship curriculum. *Med Teacher*. 2009;31:812–821.

56. Taylor D, Miflin B. Problem-based learning: Where are we now? AMEE Guide No. 36. *Med Teacher*. 2008;30:742–763.

57. Koh GCH, Khoo HE, Wong ML, et al. The effects of problem-based learning during medical school on physician competency: a systematic review. *CMAJ*. 2008;178:34–41.

58. Azer SA. Becoming a student in a PBL course: twelve tips for successful group discussion. *Med Teacher*. 2004;26:12–15.

59. Azer SA. Challenges facing PBL tutors: 12 tips for successful group facilitation. *Med Teacher*. 2005;27:676–681.

60. Azer SA. Twelve tips for creating trigger images for problem-based learning cases. *Med Teacher*. 2007;29:93–97.

61. Azer SA. Interactions between students and tutor in problem-based learning: The significance of deep learning. *Kaohsiung J Med Sci*. 2009;25:240–249.

62. Azer SA. What makes a great lecture? Use of lectures in a hybrid PBL curriculum. *Kaohsiung J Med Sci*. 2009;25:109–115.

63. Michaelson LK, Parmelee DX, McMahon KK. In: Michaelson LK, Parmelee DX, McMahon KK, eds. *Team-based learning for health professions education: A guide to using small groups for improving learning*. Sterling: Stylus Publishing; 2007.

64. Michaelson LK, Sweet M, Parmelee DX. *Team-based learning: Small group learning's next big step*. San Francisco: Jossey-Bass; 2009.

9

65. Graffam B. Active learning in medical education: Strategies for beginning implementation. *Med Teacher.* 2007;29:38–42.

66. Mayer RE. Applying the science of learning: evidence-based principles for the design of multimedia instruction. *Am Psychol.* 2008;63:760–769.

67. Means B, Toyama Y, Murphy R, et al. *Evaluation of evidence-based practices in online learning: a meta-analysis and review of online learning studies.* US Department of Education; 2009.

68. Issenberg SB, McGaghie WC, Petrusa ER, et al. Features and uses of high-fidelity medical simulations that lead to effective learning: a BEME systematic review. *Med Teacher.* 2005;27:10–28.

69. Ziv A, Ben-David S, Ziv M. Simulation based medical education: an opportunity to learn from errors. *Med Teacher.* 2005;27:193–199.

70. Ruiz JG, Cook DA, Levinson AJ. Computer animations in medical education: a critical literature review. *Med Educ.* 2009;43:838–846.

71. Kneebone R. Simulation and transformational change: The paradox of expertise. *Acad Med.* 2009;84:954–957.

72. Epstein RM. Assessment in medical education. *N Engl J Med.* 2007;356:387–396.

73. Larsen DP, Butler AC, Roediger HL. Test-enhanced learning in medical education. *Med Educ.* 2008;42:959–966.

74. Hols-Elders W, Bloemendaal P, Bos N, et al. Twelve tips for computer-based assessment in medical education. *Med Teacher.* 2008;30:673–678.

75. Kogan JR, Holmboe ES, Hauer KE. Tools for direct observation and assessment of clinical skills of medical trainees: A systematic review. *JAMA.* 2009;302:1316–1326.

76. DeAngelis CD. Professors not professing. *JAMA.* 2004;292:1060–1061.

77. LaCombe M. High society. *CMAJ.* 2002;166:1044–1045.

78. Crites G.E, Richardson W.S, Stolfi A, et al. An evidence-based medicine and clinical decision making course was successfully integrated into a medical school's preclinical, systems-based curriculum. *Med Teacher.* (manuscript submitted).

79. Richardson WS. A teacher's dozen. *Nordic Evidence-Based Health Care Newslett.* 2001;5:167.

80. Beckman TJ. Lessons learned from a peer review of bedside teaching. *Acad Med.* 2004;79:343–346.

81. Wyer PC, Keitz SA, Hatala RM, et al, for the Evidence-Based Medicine Teaching Tips Working Group. Tips for learning and teaching EBM: Introduction to the series [Commentary]. *CMAJ.* 2004;171:347–348.

82. Barratt A, Wyer PC, Hatala RM, et al, for the Evidence-Based Medicine Teaching Tips Working Group. Tips for learners of EBM: 1. Relative risk reduction, absolute risk reduction, and number needed to treat. *CMAJ*. 2004;171:353–358.

83. Montori VM, Kleinbart J, Newman TB, et al, for the Evidence-Based Medicine Teaching Tips Working Group. Tips for learners of EBM: 2. Measures of precision (confidence intervals). *CMAJ*. 2004;171:611–615.

84. McGinn TG, Wyer PC, Newman TB, et al, for the Evidence-Based Medicine Teaching Tips Working Group. Tips for learners of EBM: 3. Measures of observer variability (kappa statistic). *CMAJ*. 2004;171:1369–1373.

85. Hatala RM, Keitz SA, Wyer PC, et al, for the Evidence-Based Medicine Teaching Tips Working Group. Tips for learners of EBM: 4. Assessing heterogeneity of primary studies in systematic reviews and whether to combine their results. *CMAJ*. 2005;172:661–665.

86. Montori VM, Wyer PC, Newman TB, et al, for the Evidence-Based Medicine Teaching Tips Working Group. Tips for learners of EBM: 5. The effect of spectrum of disease on the performance of diagnostic tests. *CMAJ*. 2005;173:385–390.

87. Richardson WS, Wilson MC, Keitz SA, et al, for the EBM Teaching Scripts Working Group. Tips for teachers of evidence-based medicine: making sense of diagnostic test results using likelihood ratios. *J Gen Intern Med*. 2008;23(1):87–92.

88. Prasad K, Jaeschke R, Wyer P, et al, for the Evidence-Based Medicine Teaching Tips Working Group. Tips for teachers of evidence-based medicine: understanding odds ratios and their relationship to risk ratios. *J Gen Intern Med*. 2008;23(5):635–640.

89. Kennedy CC, Jaeschke R, Keitz SA, et al, for the Evidence-Based Medicine Teaching Tips Working Group. Tips for teachers of evidence-based medicine: adjusting for prognostic imbalances (confounding variables) in studies on therapy or harm. *J Gen Intern Med*. 2008;23(3):337–343.

90. McGinn T, Jervis R, Wisnivesky J, et al, for the Evidence-Based Medicine Teaching Tips Working Group. Tips for teachers of evidence-based medicine: Clinical prediction rules (CPRs) and estimating pretest probability. *J Gen Intern Med*. 2008;23(8):1261–1268.

91. Lee A, Joynt GM, Ho AM, et al, for the Evidence-Based Medicine Teaching Tips Working Group. Tips for teachers of evidence-based medicine: making sense of decision analysis using a decision tree. *J Gen Intern Med*. 2009;24(5):642–648.

92. Tiberius RG. *Small group teaching: A trouble-shooting guide*. Toronto: OISE Press; 1990.

9

93. Jason H, Westberg J. *Fostering learning in small groups: A practical guide.* Philadelphia: Springer; 1996.

94. Brookfield SD, Preskill S. *Discussion as a way of teaching: Tools and techniques for democratic classrooms.* San Francisco: Jossey-Bass; 1999.

95. Maudsley G. Roles and responsibilities of the problem based learning tutor in the undergraduate medical curriculum. *BMJ.* 1999;318:657–661.

96. Jaques D, Salmon G. *Learning in groups: A handbook for face-to-face and online environments.* 4th ed. Oxford: Routledge; 2007.

97. Elwyn G, Greenhalgh T, Macfarlane F. *Groups: a guide to small group work in healthcare, management, education and research.* Oxford: Radcliffe Publishing; 2001.

98. Exley K, Dennick R. *Small group teaching: Tutorials, seminars, and beyond.* London: Routledge Falmer; 2004.

99. McCrorie P. *Teaching and leading small groups. Understanding Medical Education Booklet Series.* Edinburgh: ASME; 2007.

Appendix: Glossary

Terms you are likely to encounter in your clinical reading

Absolute risk reduction (ARR). See Treatment effects.

Allocation concealment. Occurs when the person who is enrolling a participant into a clinical trial is unaware whether the next participant to be enrolled will be allocated to the intervention or control group.

Case–control study. A study which involves identifying patients who have the outcome of interest (cases) and control patients without the same outcome, and looking back to see if they had the exposure of interest.

Case series. A report on a series of patients with an outcome of interest. No control group is involved.

Clinical practice guideline. A systematically developed statement designed to assist clinician and patient decisions about appropriate healthcare for specific clinical circumstances.

Cohort study. Involves identification of two groups (cohorts) of patients, one that received the exposure of interest, and one that did not, and following these cohorts forward for the outcome of interest.

Confidence interval (CI). Quantifies the uncertainty in measurement. It is usually reported as 95% CI, which is the range of values within which we can be 95% sure that the true value for the whole population lies. For example, for an NNT of 10 with a 95% CI of 5–15, we would have 95% confidence that the true NNT value lies between 5 and 15.

Control event rate (CER). See Treatment effects.

Cost–benefit analysis. Assesses whether the cost of an intervention is worth the benefit by measuring both in the same units; monetary units are usually used.

Cost-effectiveness analysis. Measures the net cost of providing an intervention as well as the outcomes obtained. Outcomes are reported in a single unit of measurement.

Cost minimization analysis. If health effects are known to be equal, only costs are analyzed and the least costly alternative is chosen.

Cost–utility analysis. Converts health effects into personal preferences (or utilities) and describes how much it costs for some additional quality gain (e.g., cost per additional quality-adjusted life-year, or QALY).

Crossover study design. The administration of two or more experimental therapies one after the other in a specified or random order to the same group of patients.

Cross-sectional study. The observation of a defined population at a single point in time or time interval. Exposure and outcome are determined simultaneously.

Decision analysis (or clinical decision analysis). The application of explicit, quantitative methods that quantify prognoses, treatment effects, and patient values in order to analyze a decision under conditions of uncertainty.

Event rate. The proportion of patients in a group in whom the event is observed. Thus, if out of 100 patients, the event is observed in 27, the event rate is 0.27. Control event rate (CER) and experimental event rate (EER) are used to refer to this rate in control and experimental groups of patients, respectively. The patient expected event rate (PEER) refers to the rate of events we'd expect in a patient who received no treatment or conventional treatment. See Treatment effects.

Evidence-based healthcare. Extends the application of the principles of evidence-based medicine (see below) to all professions associated with healthcare, including purchasing and management.

Evidence-based medicine. The conscientious, explicit and judicious use of current best evidence in making decisions about the care of individual patients. The practice of evidence-based medicine requires the integration of individual clinical expertise with the best available external clinical evidence from systematic research and our patient's unique values and circumstances.

Experimental event rate (EER). See Treatment effects.

Incidence. The proportion of new cases of the target disorder in the population at risk during a specified time interval.

Inception cohort. A group of patients who are assembled near the onset of the target disorder.

Intention-to-treat analysis. A method of analysis for randomized trials in which all patients randomly assigned to one of the treatments are analyzed together, regardless of whether or not they completed or received that treatment, in order to preserve randomization.

Likelihood ratio (LR). The likelihood that a given test result would be expected in a patient with the target disorder compared with the likelihood that that same result would be expected in a patient without the target disorder. See below for calculations.

Meta-analysis. A systematic review that uses quantitative methods to synthesize and summarize the results.

N-of-1 trials. In such trials, the patient undergoes pairs of treatment periods organized so that one period involves the use of the experimental treatment and the other involves the use of an alternate or placebo therapy. The patient and physician are blinded, if possible, and outcomes are monitored. Treatment periods are replicated until the clinician and patient are convinced that the treatments are definitely different or definitely not different.

Negative predictive value. Proportion of people with a negative test who are free of the target disorder. See also Likelihood ratio.

Number needed to treat (NNT). The inverse of the absolute risk reduction and the number of patients that need to be treated to prevent one bad outcome. See Treatment effects.

Odds. A ratio of the number of people incurring an outcome event to the number of people who don't have an event.

Odds ratio (OR). The ratio of the odds of having the target disorder in the experimental group relative to the odds in favor of having the target disorder in the control group (in cohort studies or systematic reviews) or the odds in favor of being exposed in participants with the target disorder divided by the odds in favor of being exposed in control participants (without the target disorder). See below for calculations.

Patient expected event rate. See Treatment effects.

Overview. See Systematic review.

Positive predictive value. Proportion of people with a positive test who have the target disorder. See also Likelihood ratio.

Post-test odds. The odds that the patient has the target disorder after the test is carried out (calculated as: pre-test odds × likelihood ratio).

Post-test probability. The proportion of patients with that particular test result who have the target disorder (post-test odds/[1 + post-test odds]).

Pre-test odds. The odds that the patient has the target disorder before the test is carried out (pre-test probability/[1 − pre-test probability]).

Pre-test probability/prevalence. The proportion of people with the target disorder in the population at risk at a specific time (point prevalence) or time interval (period prevalence) See also Likelihood ratio.

Randomization (or random allocation). Method analogous to tossing a coin to assign patients to treatment groups (the experimental treatment is assigned if the coin lands "heads" and a conventional, "control" or "placebo" treatment is given if the coin lands "tails").

Randomized controlled clinical trial (RCT). Participants are randomly allocated into an experimental group or a control group and followed over time for the variables/outcomes of interest.

Relative risk reduction (RRR). See Treatment effects.

Risk ratio (RR). The ratio of the risk of the outcome event in the treated group (EER) to the risk of the event in the control group (CER) – used in randomized trials and cohort studies: RR = EER/ CER. Also called relative risk.

Sensitivity. Proportion of people with the target disorder who have a positive test result. It is used to assist in assessing and selecting a diagnostic test/sign/symptom. See also Likelihood ratio.

SnNout. When a sign/test/symptom has a high Sensitivity, a Negative result can help rule out the diagnosis. For example, the sensitivity of a history of ankle swelling for diagnosing ascites is 93%; therefore if a person does not have a history of ankle swelling, it is highly unlikely that the person has ascites.

Specificity. Proportion of people without the target disorder who have a negative test result. It is used to assist in assessing and selecting a diagnostic test/sign/symptom. See also Likelihood ratio.

SpPin. When a sign/test/symptom has a high Specificity, a Positive result can help to rule in the diagnosis. For example, the specificity of a fluid wave for diagnosing ascites is 92%; therefore if a person does have a fluid wave, it rules in the diagnosis of ascites.

Systematic review. A summary of the clinical literature that uses explicit methods to perform a comprehensive literature search and critical appraisal of individual studies and that may use appropriate statistical techniques to combine these valid studies when appropriate. The statistical technique for pooling studies is called a meta-analysis.

Treatment effects. The evidence-based journals (*Evidence Based Medicine* and *ACP Journal Club*) have achieved consensus on some terms they use to describe both the good and bad effects of therapy. We will illustrate them using a synthesis of three randomized trials in diabetes which individually showed that several years of intensive insulin therapy reduced the proportion of patients with worsening retinopathy to 13% from 38%, raised the proportion of patients with satisfactory hemoglobin A_{1c} levels to 60% from about 30%, and increased the proportion of patients with at least one episode of symptomatic hypoglycemia to 57% from 23%. Note that in each case the first number constitutes the "experimental event rate" (EER) and the second number the "control event rate" (CER). We will use the following terms and calculations to describe these effects of treatment.

When the experimental treatment reduces the probability of a bad outcome (worsening diabetic retinopathy):

RRR (relative risk reduction). The proportional reduction in rates of bad outcomes between experimental and control participants in a trial, calculated as |EER−CER|/CER, and accompanied by a 95% confidence interval (CI). In the case of worsening diabetic retinopathy, |EER−CER|/CER = |13%−38%|/38% = 66%.

ARR (absolute risk reduction). The absolute arithmetic difference in rates of bad outcomes between experimental and control participants in a trial, calculated as |EER−CER|, and accompanied by a 95% CI. In this case, |EER−CER| = 13%−38%| = 25%. (This is sometimes called the risk difference).

NNT (number needed to treat). The number of patients who need to be treated to achieve one additional favorable outcome, calculated as 1/ARR and accompanied by a 95% CI. In this case, 1/ARR = 1/25% = 4.

When the experimental treatment increases the probability of a good outcome (satisfactory hemoglobin A_{1c} levels):

RBI (relative benefit increase). The proportional increase in rates of good outcomes between experimental and control patients in a trial, calculated as |EER − CER|/CER, and accompanied by a 95% confidence interval (CI). In the case of satisfactory hemoglobin A_{1c} levels, |EER − CER|/CER = |60% − 30%|/30% = 100%.

ABI (absolute benefit increase). The absolute arithmetic difference in rates of good outcomes between experimental and control patients in a trial, calculated as |EER − CER|, and accompanied by a 95% confidence interval (CI). In the case of satisfactory hemoglobin A_{1c} levels, |EER − CER| = |60% − 30%| = 30%.

NNT (number needed to treat). The number of patients who need to be treated to achieve one additional good outcome, calculated as 1/ARR and accompanied by a 95% CI. In this case, 1/ARR = 1/30% = 3.

When the experimental treatment increase the probability of a bad outcome (episodes of hypoglycemia):

RRI (relative risk increase). The proportional increase in rates of bad outcomes between experimental and control patients in a trial, calculated as |EER − CER|/CER, and accompanied by a 95% confidence interval (CI). In the case of hypoglycemic episodes, |EER − CER|/CER = |57% − 23%|/23% = 148%. (RRI is also used in assessing the impact of "risk factors" for disease.)

ARI (absolute risk increase). The absolute arithmetic difference in rates of bad outcomes between experimental and control patients in a trial, calculated as |EER − CER|, and accompanied by a 95% confidence interval (CI). In the case of hypoglycemic episodes, |EER − CER| = |57% − 23%| = 34%. (ARI is also used in assessing the impact of "risk factors" for disease.)

NNH (number needed to harm). The number of patients who, if they received the experimental treatment, would result in one additional patient being harmed, compared with patients who received the control treatment, calculated as 1/ARR and accompanied by a 95% CI. In this case, 1/ARR = 1/34% = 3.

Table A.1 Treatment effects				
Occurrence of diabetic retinopathy at 5 years among insulin-dependent diabetics	Relative risk reduction	Absolute risk reduction	Number needed to treat (NNT)	
Usual insulin regimen (CER)	Intensive insulin regimen (EER)	$\dfrac{\|EER-CER\|}{CER}$	$\|EER-CER\|$	1/ARR
38%	13%	$\|13\% - 38\%\|/38\%$ $= 68\%$	$\|13\% - 38\%\|$ $= 25\%$	1/25% $= 4$ patients

How to calculate LRs

We can assume that there are four possible groups of patients, as indicated (a,b,c,d) in Table A.2.

Table A.2 Test annually		Target disorder		
		Present	Absent	
Diagnostic test result	+	a	b	a+b
	−	c	d	c+d
		a+c	b+d	a+b+c+d

From these we can determine the *sensitivity* and *specificity* as follows:

Sensitivity $= a/(a + c)$
Specificity $= d/(b + d)$

We can consider the calculation of the likelihood ratio for a positive test in a couple of ways:

1. We can consider how likely is a positive test in someone with the disease?

$= a/(a + c)$

We also need to consider how likely is a positive test result in someone without the disease?

$= b/(b + d)$

And, how likely is this test result to occur in someone with compared to someone without the disease?

$= (a/(a + c))/(b/(b + d))$

2. We can use sensitivity and specificity to calculate the likelihood ratio for a positive test result (LR+):

LR+ = sensitivity/(1 − specificity)

$$= [a/(a+c)] \div [b/(b+d)]$$

Similarly, we can calculate the likelihood ratio for a negative test result (LR−):

LR− = (1 − sensitivity)/specificity

$$= [c/(a+c)] \div [d/(b+d)]$$

Positive predictive value = $a/(a+b)$

Negative predictive value = $d/(c+d)$

Pre-test probability = $(a+c)/(a+b+c+d)$.

Sample calculation

Suppose you have a patient with anemia and a serum ferritin of 60 mmol/L. You come across a systematic review* of serum ferritin as a diagnostic test for iron deficiency anemia, with the results summarized as in Table A.3.

These results indicate that 90% of the patients with iron deficiency anemia have a positive test result (serum ferritin <65 mmol/L). This is known as the sensitivity and is calculated as:

Sensitivity = $a/(a+c)$ = 731/809 = 90%

Table A.3 Test annually		Target disorder (iron deficiency anemia)		
		Present	Absent	
Diagnostic test result (serum ferritin)	+ (<65 mmol/L)	731 a	270 b	1001 a+b
	− (≥65 mmol/L)	c 78	d 1500	c+d 1578
		a+c 809	b+d 1770	a+b+c+d 2579

---

* Guyatt GH, Oxman AD, Ali M, et al. Laboratory diagnosis of iron-deficiency anemia: an overview. J Gen Intern Med 1992; 7 (2): 145–153. Erratum in: J Gen Intern Med 1992; 7 (4): 423.

The results also show that 85% of patients who do not have iron deficiency anemia have a negative test result. This is referred to as the specificity, calculated as:

Specificity $= d/(b + d) = 1500/1770 = 85\%$

From these the positive and negative likelihood ratios can be determined:

LR+ = sensitivity/

$(1 - specificity) = 90\%/15\% = 6$

LR− = (1 − sensitivity)/

specificity $= 10\%/85\% = 0.12$

Thus, from your calculation of LR+ you determine that your patient's positive test result would be about six times as likely to be seen in someone with iron deficiency anemia than in someone without the disorder.

Calculation of odds ratio/relative risk

Calculation of odds ratio/relative risk for the use of trimethoprim-sulfamethoxazole prophylaxis in cirrhosis:

Table A.4 Odds ratio/relative risk

	Adverse event occurs (infectious complication)	Adverse event doesn't occur (no infectious complication)	Totals
Exposed to treatment (experimental)	1	29	30
	a	b	a+b
Not exposed to treatment (control)	9	21	30
	c	d	c+d
Totals	10	50	60
	a+c	b+d	a+b +c+d

CER = c/(c + d) = 0.30
EER = a/(a + b) = 0.033
Control event odds = c/d = 0.43
Experimental event odds = a/b = 0.034
Relative risk = EER/CER = 0.11
Relative odds = odds ratio = (a/b)/(c/d) = ad/bc = 0.08

Note that risks = odds/(1 + odds) and odds = risk/(1 − risk). We used the second equation in the description of post-test odds and probabilities above. We convert pre-test probabilities to pre-test odds to allow us to multiply this by the likelihood ratio. We then used the first equation to convert from post-test odds to post-test probability.

Index

Note: Page numbers followed by *b* indicate boxes, *f* indicate figures and *t* indicate tables.